Flying Monkeys, Floating Stones

Flying Monkeys, Floating Stones

*Wisdom Tales from the Ramayana
for Modern Yogis*

Zo Newell, PhD

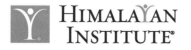

HIMALAYAN
INSTITUTE®

HONESDALE, PENNSYLVANIA USA

The Himalayan Institute Press
952 Bethany Turnpike
Honesdale, PA 18431 USA

www.HimalayanInstitute.org

© 2021 by Himalayan International Institute of Yoga Science
and Philosophy of the U.S.A.®

Printed in the United States of America

25 24 23 22 21   1 2 3 4 5

ISBN-13: 978-0-89389-283-8 (paper)

Photos by Andrea Killam
Author photo by Greg Butler
Models: Judy Moulton and Shawn Laster

Library of Congress Control Number: 2021904229

♾ This paper meets the requirements of ANSI/NISO Z39-48-1992
(Permanence of Paper).

With gratitude to all my teachers.

Contents

Preface

When I was a child, I was blessed with a yoga teacher who was a storyteller. Sri Brahmananda Sarasvati taught that the practice of yoga leads us from ignorance to wisdom and from false identification with our limitations to the realization of our true nature as eternal. He often used tales from Indian mythology to teach his students about human relationships and the spiritual path. He approached the *Ramayana,* the epic story of Lord Rama and his beloved wife, Sita, as a parable about yoga, with Sita and Rama's separation symbolizing the division between distracted consciousness and the Self, the object of meditation. He emphasized Sita and Rama's symbolic meaning as elements of the human psyche. To me, at that time, Sita was an ideal to emulate—loyal and brave, and persistent in her determination to reunite with Rama— but more an abstraction than a person.

Many years later, I was in India visiting places associated with Meher Baba. Near his home at Pimpalgaon, Maharashtra, is a spot known as Happy Valley, or Sita Kund. Rama, Sita, and Lakshmana were said to have sojourned there, living for several days in one of the caves. This part of India is dry and arid, like the semidesert of Southern California. When you travel, your clothing, spectacles, and nasal passages quickly become coated with a fine, earth-scented dust. We had driven on bad roads, through noisy, diesel-laced traffic, to reach the site, a deep crater in the earth, its sides covered with green trees, rocks, and caves.

We stepped onto a long stone staircase, its top step level with the dry ground, and descended gradually below the surface, toward the scent of water. The air became fresher and cleaner; the sounds of traffic died away. It was as if we were leaving the modern world for some eternal, mythical realm. At the bottom, the air felt cool and smelled of wet rock. The guide led us to a place where silver streams of water splashed musically down the dark rock face. "Sita Kund," he said: Sita's Pool. In this spot, Rama had shot an arrow into the earth so she could bathe. For some reason this astonished me. "Sita?" I said, probably sounding a little incredulous. He nodded. "Sita," he replied firmly. And suddenly she was real to me—as real as the landscape. A woman like me, Sita had climbed down, hot and dusty, and stepped gratefully into this same pool where I now dipped my toe. She smelled the fresh, cool air and heard the plink of drops falling down the rocks, just as I did. What I experienced now, she had felt all those ages ago.

In this book I present stories and images from the *Ramayana* through art and asana. It is my hope that these stories will speak to you—through your body and your senses as well as your mind—and allow you a glimpse of their reality. Following my teacher's approach, I invite the reader to approach the stories and their characters as symbols for the practice of yoga: Sita is the intelligence "kidnapped" by Ravana (the ego), and she must be reunited with Rama (the Self) in meditation through the actions of Hanuman and the animal army (asana and pranayama practice). But let us remember, symbols are living things— the outward, visible signs of an inner, dynamic process. By marrying the stories and symbols to specific asanas, and by engaging with them through writing and imagination, I hope they will become as real for you as Sita did for me that day in Happy Valley.

How to Use This Book

In my own practice, I find writing and journaling to be tremendously helpful tools. For this kind of writing, I recommend the method that Natalie Goldberg presents in her classic, *Writing Down the Bones*: Choose a writing prompt—perhaps some aspect of the story or of your experience with the related asana. Decide how long you will write, and stick to it. Keep your hand moving; don't edit yourself. Just write it, and be as specific as you can (a magnolia, not a tree).

Set a timer. Stop when it rings, even in the middle of a sentence. If you run out of things to say before the designated time, keep your hand moving. Trust that there is something behind that apparent lack of thoughts. Write about what's in front of you. You can write: "Writing, writing, no ideas, bright room, wood floor, blue table, purple yoga mat . . ." It doesn't matter. You are still directing the movements of your mind. The point is not only to let thoughts arise and observe them but also to channel those thoughts—order them, shape them.

It can be interesting to begin with a very short-timed writing, two to three minutes, in which you observe yourself: your thoughts, your breath, your emotions (which, in yoga, count as part of your mind), and your body at the beginning of your practice. Write a few words about what you observe. For example, "Left knee stiff, breath shallow, more in right nostril, left shoulder tight, mind distracted, like starting new things, chiropractor??" Now choose your pose, do the pose, choose your writing prompt, and go!—say, for ten minutes. At the end of your practice, take a couple of minutes to observe your body and breath again, and write down what you find. Is there any difference in your breath, your shoulder, the quality of your thoughts? Are you still thinking of becoming a chiropractor (or consulting one, or whatever you meant by that)?

This kind of journaling is an excellent way to begin observing your thoughts and their qualities. You may find that the very act of observation begins to loosen their habitual patterns and free your mind. Over time, notice what themes and realizations emerge. Through this process, my teacher would say, you reveal the *Ramayana* hidden within you.

For people who do not enjoy writing—don't force yourself! You may still enjoy using some of the questions and reflections included in each story for your own inner exploration.

Introduction

Indian literature embraces a genre known as *itihasa*, "it so happened." This class of stories includes the great epics the *Ramayana* and the *Mahabharata*, as well as the vast body of wisdom literature known as the Puranas. *Itihasa* is often rendered in English as "mythology," but this term can confuse English speakers because we have so devalued our own mythic traditions that we now understand "myth" to mean something that is not evidence-based, something not true. Here, I use "myth" to mean stories that are psychologically true, whether or not they can be documented as having happened, and that help us find our way in a world that is often confusing.

The *Ramayana* narrates the life of Rama, prince of Ayodhya and an incarnation of the preserver, Lord Vishnu, who returns to earth when humankind's need is greatest. The key events are Rama's exile and wandering in the forest with his wife, Sita (an incarnation of Vishnu's eternal consort, Lakshmi Devi), and his brother Lakshmana; Sita's abduction and captivity by Ravana, the demon king of Lanka; Sita's rescue by Rama's army; Sita's trial by fire to verify her purity after her abduction by Ravana; and the triumphant return of Rama, Sita, and Lakshmana to Ayodhya, where Rama is installed as king, and Sita—again the subject of doubts about her purity—is sent to live in the forest, gives birth to twin sons, and returns to the divine realm.

The story's reputed composer was Valmiki, a retired outlaw turned poet-sage who lived and wrote in the northern part of India in ancient times. However, the story's life far exceeds Valmiki's, or any, written text. It flourishes in multiple languages and cultural variants, in folk song, dance, and drama; as a hugely popular Indian television series; in graphic novels; and in film. There are feminist interpretations and nationalist interpretations. Aside from Valmiki's version, one of the most widely venerated retellings is Tulsidas's sixteenth-century *Ramcharitmanas*. The *Adhyatma Ramayana*, one of Tulsidas's sources and my teacher's inspiration, emphasizes Rama's divine nature and assures spiritual liberation to anyone who hears or repeats his story with devotion. I have drawn on this version for many of the stories here. The thing to remember is that just as everyone has his or her individual path to the divine, each of us provides the setting for our inner *Ramayana* to unfold.

Omnipresent though Rama is in India, physical evidence for his reign is sparse. Some doubt that he ever lived on earth. Some champions of the story's historicity point to the undoubted existence of a submerged causeway connecting India and Sri Lanka, still visible in NASA photographs and passable by foot until the 1400s; but that bridge is estimated to be one million years old, while Rama is believed to have lived several thousand years ago.

Rama is one of the most beloved aspects of the Divine in all of Indian history. His presence pervades India's culture. Gandhi died with his name on his lips. People repeat his name, inscribe it on their garments and jewelry, sing it, celebrate it. He and his beloved Sita are revered as the perfect man and woman, their marriage an ideal for all to emulate. He also embodies the ideal of *dharma raja*, the ruler who values right action and the common good above individual concerns. Mothers pray to have a son like Rama, a daughter like Sita. Historical evidence aside, their story is true in the sense that myths are true spiritually and psychologically.

The Story

Rama was born to Dasharatha, the king of Ayodhya, in the king's old age. Through divine intervention, Dasharatha's three wives gave birth to four sons all on the same day. Rama was the firstborn and Dasharatha's obvious successor. Everyone, including his brothers and stepmothers, loved Rama and looked forward to his becoming king. However, when Dasharatha decided to retire and pass the throne to Rama, suddenly the mind of the second wife, Kaikeyi, was poisoned by jealousy on behalf of her own son, Bharata.

Many years before, as a young warrior-queen, Kaikeyi had saved Dasharatha's life on the battlefield. Grateful, he promised her two boons, payable at any time. Now Kaikeyi, at the instigation of her servant Manthara, called in this favor. She demanded that Dasharatha seat Bharata on the throne and exile Rama to the forest for fourteen years.

Dasharatha was shocked, horrified, heartbroken—but a king's word is not to be broken, and he had to bow to Kaikeyi's request. Sadly, and with deep bitterness, Dasharatha broke the news to the people: Bharata, not Rama, would succeed him.

Bharata was stunned. He knew well that Rama was the born ruler and that he was not. Rama, however, accepted his father's decision with equanimity. Accompanied by Sita and his brother Lakshmana, he exchanged his royal robes for simple traveling clothes and set forth into exile. The trio soon found refuge with forest yogis. They stopped first at Sage Bharadvaja's hermitage; Bharadvaja directed them to the Dandaka Forest, near modern Nasik, on the banks of the Godavari River. Here, in a place still known as Panchavati, they built a hut in a grove of five banyan trees (*pancha* means "five;" *vati* means "banyan") and lived a simple, happy life.

In Indian cosmology, the universe is governed by three main principles, or deities: Brahma, the creator; Vishnu, the preserver; and Shiva, the destroyer. From time to time, when *dharma* (cosmic order) is threatened, Vishnu takes birth in an appropriate form to set things right. The reason Lord Vishnu had incarnated as Rama was to stop the demon Ravana from wreaking havoc on the entire earth, beginning with the yogis in the Dandaka Forest. For his own reasons, Ravana hoped to lure Rama into a confrontation. When he learned of Rama's presence in the very forest he was despoiling, Ravana saw his chance. He kidnapped Sita and flew off with her to his island stronghold, Lanka.

Rama and Lakshmana searched everywhere. They found allies in the warrior bird Jatayu and in Hanuman, the *vanar* (monkey) general and superhero. Aided by an army of bears and monkeys, Rama built a magical bridge of floating stones, crossed it, and won the battle of Lanka, in which Ravana was killed and Sita was rescued. But before she could rejoin Rama, she had to undergo a trial by fire to establish publicly, beyond a doubt, that her purity had not been compromised by Ravana during her captivity. Sita entered the fire, but she was not burned. After she emerged unharmed from the fire, she and Rama were reunited and returned home, triumphant, to Ayodhya. But a problem soon arose. Because Sita had lived in the palace of another king, evil-minded people questioned her fidelity to Rama, despite her trial by fire in Lanka. These insinuations intensified when Sita became pregnant.

Rama was forced to send Sita away, back to the forest. Sita had her babies, twin boys, in Valmiki's ashram—the same Valmiki who composed the story of Rama and Sita. Without Sita, Rama felt incomplete. Eventually he met his sons, learned her whereabouts, and invited all of them to return to Ayodhya. When they arrived at Rama's palace, Sita, the daughter of Mother Earth, was asked once again to publicly attest to her purity, so she called out to Mother Earth to take her back. The earth opened, and Mother Earth rose up to receive her. Rama was heartbroken without her. After ruling for many years, he, too, left his body by walking into the river Sarayu. Rama and Sita were reunited beyond time and space, to return in a future age.

At this point we, the audience, are aghast, and may be thinking harsh thoughts about Rama. But remember: Rama is Vishnu, the preserver; Sita is his consort, Lakshmi. They come to earth from time to time, always together, and then they return to heaven to rest and enjoy themselves between incarnations. All of this was part of the divine game. But one thing is clear: Rama and Sita are united now in their eternal abode, and within our hearts and psyches as well.

Interpreting Myth

Scholars of religious studies propose an understanding of myth as "meaning-making narrative," a way to make sense of a world or circumstance that does not seem to make sense. It might be a personal dilemma: Should I marry this person, embrace this career change, move to another country, choose chemotherapy or alternative medicine? Or a collective challenge: Why is there death? How was the earth created? Through myth, collective psychology expresses itself in story, as individual psychology expresses itself in dreams. But unlike dreams, myths widen our perspective, letting us see that the story is not strictly about us and has broader, maybe even universal, importance.

Asana, too, is a valuable tool for seeing the connections between how we are on the mat and how we are in our lives. Each asana lets us observe ourselves in a particular process or situation: How do I approach the problem of, say, tight shoulders? If an action is difficult, do I trust that there is a way to make friends with the difficulty, or am I angry or frustrated? Do I look for someone to blame for my frustration? Do I feel that my body or the teacher or the pose is an enemy, or a potential friend? What narrative about myself or the universe do I tell myself in a situation of this kind? Asana and myth are twin paths to wisdom and insight. By including both in our practice, we may gain even richer insights into our individual and collective psyches.

My teacher Sri Brahmananda Sarasvati ("Guruji"), who had trained as a psychiatrist, explained that if understood psychologically, the characters in a myth are symbols, aspects of our unconscious minds. Reflecting on those characters' choices and their consequences can provide insight into our own choices and consequences by taking us below the surface of our usual personas, relationships, and patterns of behavior. Through yoga practice, he said, we experience the battlefield within the mind, and the constant tension between constructive and destructive mental forces—*vrittis*, as the *Yoga Sutra* calls them—that channel our attention toward, or away from, the unified consciousness that we experience in the highest state of yoga, samadhi.

Guruji approached the *Ramayana* as an allegory of the individual's psyche and spiritual journey. He broke down the story's symbols like this:

Rama represents the true Self.

Sita represents our innate intelligence.

Ravana, with his ten heads, represents the self-involved ego. His heads represent the ten senses: five senses of perception, or knowledge, and five senses of action.

Dasharatha represents the divine ego, or Self-consciousness, which also has the ten (*dasha*) senses. (*Dasharatha* means "driver of ten chariots.")

The kidnapping of Sita is the misuse of intelligence by the ten-headed ego for selfish purposes; Sita's abduction is the loss of reasoning power by one who is deluded by *maya* (illusion)—the golden deer.

Hanuman, with his strong physique, celibate habits, and devotion to the Lord, represents the invincible power of yoga practice.

This is one way of interpreting this story. I encourage you to find your own meanings for the characters and events in these stories. Ask yourself how each one relates to your personal experience. Do you identify with a particular character? What challenges do the characters face? What are their solutions? What results come from their decisions? What insights do the characters and events suggest in terms of your own life?

For this book I have chosen several stories from the *Ramayana* that I find especially appealing and have linked them with related images and asanas. I have tried to suggest points for personal reflection without interpreting the stories too rigidly, because what really matters is how they and the characters resonate with each individual who encounters them.

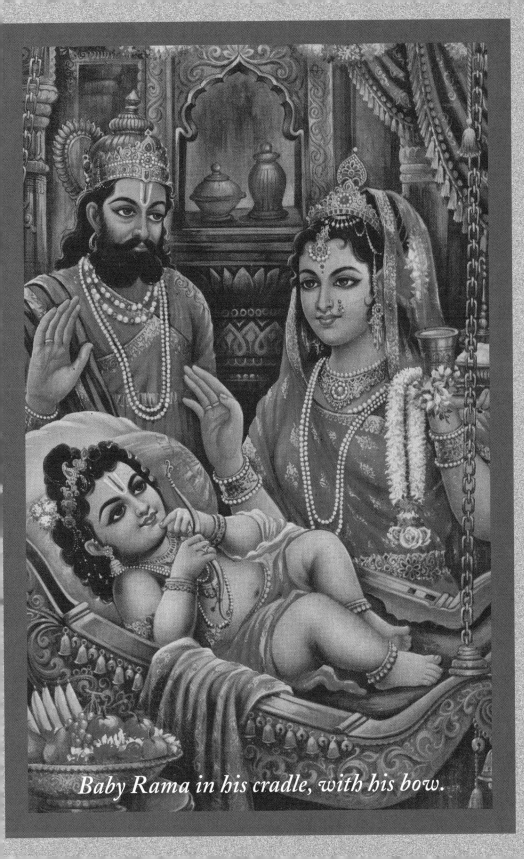

Baby Rama in his cradle, with his bow.

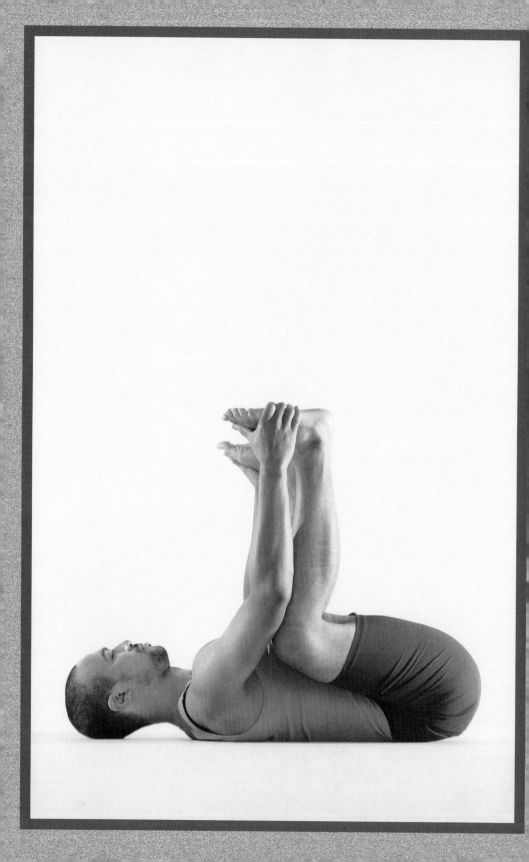

Birth of Rama

Happy Baby Pose / Ananda Balasana

Dasharatha, the king of Ayodhya, was a famous warrior and a protector of dharma. He had three brave, lovely wives, but no children, and this lack made everyone in the kingdom sad.

Even as Dasharatha longed for an heir, Bhumi Devi (Mother Earth) was praying for a champion to relieve her suffering at the hands of *rakshasas* (demons) and powerful, unscrupulous people who despoiled her body and robbed her resources for their own gain. Evil rakshasas were harassing the sages and saints in her forests, dropping filth onto their sacrificial altars, disrupting their practices, even threatening their lives.

The sacred texts tell us that when the wick of dharma burns low and evil darkens the world, Vishnu, the preserver, takes birth to set things right again. The time had come for Vishnu to return. This time he came as Dasharatha's eldest son, Rama, with a destiny to heal and protect not just Ayodhya, but Mother Earth herself.

Rama's birth was unusual. On the advice of the court sage Vasishtha, Dasharatha performed a special *yagna* (sacrifice), the *ashvamedha*. At its completion, a golden vessel filled with *payasam* (milk pudding) emerged from the sacred fire, and a voice said, "Take this home and share it with your wives."

At first he split the pudding evenly between his chief wife, Kaushalya, and his second wife, Kaikeyi. Generous Kaushalya gave half her share to the youngest queen, Sumitra; then Kaikeyi, too, gave half her share to Sumitra. All three wives became pregnant. On one happy day, Kaushalya gave birth to Rama, Kaikeyi to Bharata, and Sumitra to the twins, Lakshmana and Shatrughna. The kingdom rejoiced, and Bhumi Devi rejoiced that her champions had arrived to restore dharma and protect her body. Dasharatha and his wives loved their four children dearly, and each one had his special gift and charm, but Rama was the heart's delight of all, and everyone looked forward to the day he would be king.

Happy Baby Pose / *Ananda Balasana*

Although it is not one of the traditional poses found in older hatha yoga texts, happy baby pose (*ananda balasana*) is very popular in contemporary practice. Its benefits include opening the hips, inner thighs, chest, and shoulders; lengthening the spine; and releasing tension in the low back. It is great preparation for many seated poses. This pose resembles a reclining squat, and it offers a great alternative for people who cannot squat while bearing weight through their knees. We'll start with one side at a time, before doing the final pose (shown in the photo).

Embodying the Pose

Place a block, a folded blanket, or a bolster by your right side on which your right knee may rest, as needed. Have a yoga strap nearby in case you can't reach your foot comfortably.

To begin, lie comfortably on your back. Bend your knees. Place the soles of your feet on the floor.

Keeping the left foot on the floor, bring your right knee to your chest. Flex the right foot.

With your right hand, reach up along the outer shin to grasp the outside edge of your right foot. (If you cannot reach the outside of your foot, loop a strap over the ball of the right foot and hold the strap.) Your foot is now facing the ceiling. Keep the hips even.

Exhale. Relax your shoulders and your face.

Go slowly; notice the sensations in your leg as you draw the right knee to a right angle. Keep the foot flexed.

Rest your left hand over your left hip bone.

Exhaling, draw your right knee toward the floor, close to your ribs, as if you could place it in your armpit.

Sustaining the Pose

Keep the shoulders, chest, and tongue relaxed. Breathe!

If your knee does not reach the floor, allow the knee to rest on a prop (a block, a folded blanket, or a bolster).

Notice your foot. Do the toes point away from your body as your leg descends? You are externally rotating your thigh. What if you maintain more of an internal rotation and point the toes forward? How does this change the sensation in your right thigh?

Releasing the Pose

Finish this side by placing your right foot on the floor. Enjoy a few resting breaths with both feet on the floor.

Then begin on the opposite side (move your props to the left). Place your right foot on the floor and repeat the sequence with your left side.

Finish with a few resting breaths. Notice the difference in sensations between the two sides.

Final Step

For the final step, grasp both feet with your hands or straps and evenly draw both knees down toward the armpits, like a happy baby in her crib. Don't force it; be playful.

Babies love to play with their feet! In this pose, recapture the sheer joy and fascination of lying on your back and discovering your legs, toes, shoulders, and back.

For three days, make ananda balasana your first pose of the day. How does starting your day with a playful, open, innocent posture like this affect what comes afterward?

Reflection

In this story, a divine child, Rama—a symbol of hope and optimism—is born to the old king who has mastered control of his senses.

Rama's adventures in the world are the subject of the *Ramayana*, "Rama's journey," but we can also understand Rama's story as an allegory of our own lives and bodies. My teacher used to say that the Divine is ready to be born in us all the time; psychologically, avatars and other deities represent potentials waiting to be realized. Mythological stories and the characters in them are symbols for parts of ourselves.

Each of us is potentially Dasharatha, the commander of ten chariots. The ten chariots are our five senses of perception and five senses of action, which connect our intelligence with the physical world. The *Katha Upanishad* famously uses the image of the body as a chariot pulled by the horses of our senses along the paths of sense objects, with *atman* (soul) as the rider, *buddhi* (intelligence) as the driver, and *manas* (mind) as the reins. So Dasharatha is one who controls the mind and senses—a yogi.

Kaushalya means "skill"; Dasharatha's first wife, or attribute, is the skill to keep the mind steady on the Self and not let it be sidetracked by the senses. *Ashva* means "now, the present moment"; *medha* means "purification." *Ashvamedha* means "purifying the mind of all distractions and being present in the now." *Rama* means "one who gives happiness"; some interpreters add that *ra* means "radiance, light," and *ma* means "in me." When Dasharatha performs the ashvamedha sacrifice and shares the results with Kaushalya, the child Rama—inner radiance and joy—is conceived. When we control our mind and senses in meditation—focusing on internal reality and renouncing external claims—the divine potential within manifests: a happy baby is born. The *Bhagavad Gita* (2:50) says, *yoga karmasu kaushalam*, "yoga is skill in action." You could say that when our mind-body complex acts skillfully, we are in a state of yoga; we become en-light-ened. This is the inner meaning of Rama's birth.

However, remember that Rama is accompanied by three other qualities, represented by Dasharatha's other sons: Lakshmana (mindfulness, awareness) and Shatrughna (one who has no enemies), the sons of Sumitra (good friend); and Bharata (all talents), the son of

Kaikeyi (one who appears outwardly unpleasant but whose inner effect is deeply beneficial, like a bitter medicine).

In each of us, no matter our age, there is a "divine child" ready to be born in the form of inspiration, creative energy, or a new, unconditioned experience of the world.

Consider the characters in this story as aspects of your own psyche. What is born of your skillful efforts to control your mind and senses? What about your own qualities of mindfulness, friendliness, and talent? How have you grown through practices or experiences that seemed bitter at first?

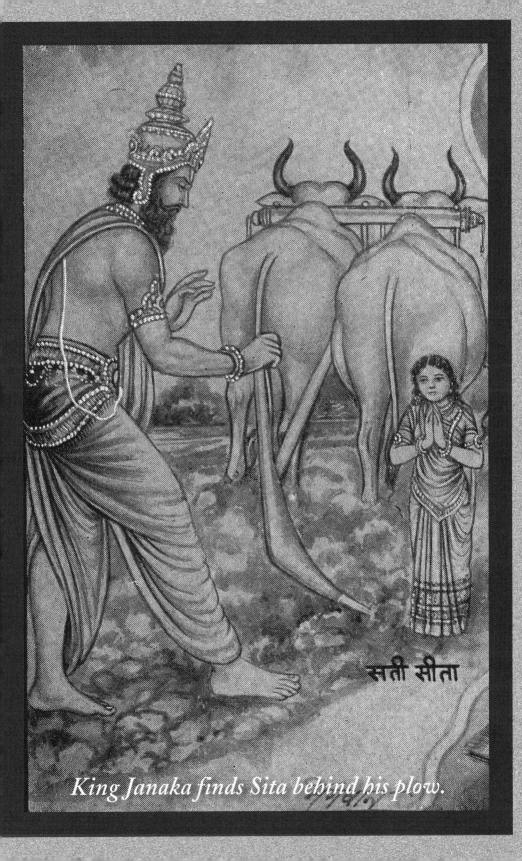

सती सीता

King Janaka finds Sita behind his plow.

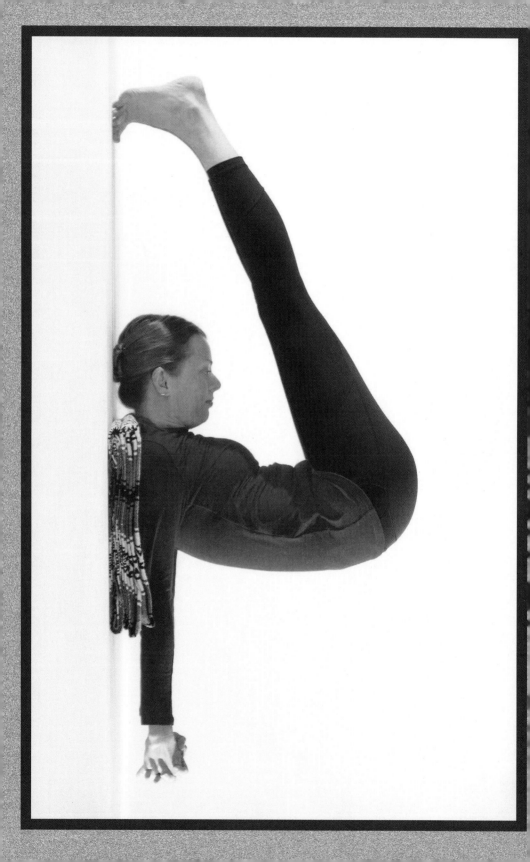

Birth of Sita

Plow Pose / Halasana

When Lord Vishnu took a human birth as Rama, the goddess Lakshmi Devi became his beloved Sita. Vishnu and Lakshmi are eternal consorts. As preserver of the universe, Vishnu assumes the role of a ruler; Lakshmi is not only his queen but the *shakti*, the power, by which he rules, upholding the world and protecting dharma. As Sita, she was born as the daughter of King Janaka and Bhumi Devi, the earth goddess.

King Janaka was a *karma yogi*, one who follows the path of service, as well as a sage. Janaka's care for his people included care for the land, and he worked the fields like any farmer. One day when he was plowing he spied something moving in the furrow he had just plowed. Afraid he might have disturbed the habitat of some small animal, he stopped and looked. No, not an animal. This small creature was not furry. King Janaka bent down and, in wonder, lifted a beautiful baby girl from the furrow (*seet*) his plow had drawn in the earth. Her large, solemn eyes regarded him calmly. "Hello, daughter," said King Janaka. The baby smiled. "You will be Sita," he told her, "because you were born in a seet."

As the daughter of Mother Earth, Sita represents the physical dimension of the universe, *prakriti*, just as Rama personifies consciousness, *purusha*. This entire creation, the sages say, springs from the love play between these two principles. To say that Sita was born from a furrow of the earth is another way of saying that we come to understand our own spiritual nature through the medium of the body.

When Sita grew up, King Janaka held a huge festival, a *svayamvara*, for her to choose her own husband. Of course, she chose Rama—but that is another story.

Plow Pose / *Halasana*

This inversion is an intermediate-to-advanced pose. It is closely related to shoulderstand (*salamba sarvangasana*). The many benefits of the plow pose include stimulating the internal organs and relieving stress. Along with the full plow pose (with blankets, as shown in the photo), I have included several modifications and one variation: reclining upward-facing head-to-knee pose (*supta paschimottanasana*), which is safer for practitioners needing to avoid inversion due to neck, eye, or shoulder issues.

Full Pose

Embodying the Pose

To begin, gather two or three blankets that are tightly woven wool or cotton, not fluffy. Fold these blankets to the same width as your mat, and stack them on top of each other on your mat, with the smooth edges aligned. (On the edge with a fringe, keep the fringe out of your way by tucking it into the blankets.) During the asana, these blankets will lift your shoulders in order to protect your neck and keep your chin from jamming into your chest.

Next, create a lift to sit on by placing a block, a bolster, or a thickly folded blanket where the smooth edges are. Sit on this lift with your back facing the blanket stack.

Lie back on the blanket stack with your shoulders two to three inches from the edges of the blankets where the fringe has been tucked in. The back of your head, not your shoulders, should be on the floor. (When your legs lift, your weight will shift in the direction of your head; if you are too close to the edge of the blankets, your shoulders will slide off.)

Be sure you are *not* resting your body's weight on C7 (the prominent vertebra at the base of the neck). Keep your eyes open throughout the asana, to reduce pressure in the eyes.

Place your arms at your sides, palms down.

Press your upper arms toward the floor and slide your shoulder blades down your back toward your feet.

Exhaling, bend your knees and bring them to your chest.

Now bend your elbows, place your hands on your back, and, inhaling, swing your legs up until your torso is as close to perpendicular to the floor as possible.

Interlace your fingers, palm-to-palm, and draw your arms away from your head. From that action, draw weight into the upper part of your shoulder blades.

Exhaling, lower your feet to the floor behind your head. Keep your knees straight and your torso as close to perpendicular to the floor as you can.

Modifications

If your back body or hamstrings are too tight to take your feet to the floor behind your head, consider taking your feet to blocks, to the seat of a chair, or to a wall (in which case, you will set up with the crown of your head facing the wall).

Having your feet rest on the floor makes this an intermediate-to-advanced pose. If you are a beginner, start with plenty of support and decrease the height as your flexibility increases.

Sustaining the Pose

Walk your hands further down your back, toward your shoulder blades; keeping your elbows closely aligned with your outer ribs, press into your upper back and slide your sternum toward your chin.

Soften your gaze and turn your eyes toward your breastbone.

Lift the inner thighs to lengthen your side waist.

Keep your feet on the floor and lift the thighbones toward the ceiling. Breathe. Once you are in the pose, do not turn your head.

Does your breathing feel restricted in this pose? Notice if you are tightening your throat or tensing your eyes. Relax your throat. Soften your gaze.

Breathe as fully as you can, not only in the upper part of the lungs. Feel the breath moving even in the back body. Feel how much space you have!

Releasing the Pose

To come out, walk your feet toward your head. Continue to support your back with your hands, then bend your knees and roll your spine down, vertebra by vertebra, to the floor.

Exhaling, roll to your right side. Stay for several breaths until you fully relax.

Finally, take your left hand to the floor and lift yourself back to a seated position.

What does this pose reveal about how you handle restrictions or limitations? Do you push through, or let your breath guide your capacity at each stage of the pose?

Cautions

Avoid this pose if you are menstruating, if you have neck or shoulder problems, or if it creates pressure in the eyes. Be sure you are not resting your body's weight on C7 (the prominent vertebra at the base of the neck). Once you are in the pose, do not turn your head.

Variation: Reclining Upward-Facing Head-to-Knee Pose /
Supta Paschimottanasana

If you must avoid inversions due to neck, shoulder, or eye issues, you may be able to practice *supta paschimottanasana* as a safe alternative. You will still experience a satisfying stretch in your back body and receive the benefits of plow pose.

Embodying the Pose

Lie on your back, with your arms alongside the body, palms down. Lift your legs, and draw your feet over your head toward the floor or to the height appropriate for your comfort. Keep your shoulder blades on the floor. Bring your hands to your feet.

Releasing the Pose

To come out, return your arms alongside the body, leave your head on the mat, bend your knees, and roll out of the position until your feet are flat on the floor. Breathe and relax.

Reflection

In this story, Sita, the divine feminine, emerges when a sage digs beneath the surface.

King Janaka, caring for his physical environment, discovers the goddess. When you nurture your body-mind through the sustained, focused practice of asana, pranayama, and meditation, what does your attention turn up? Maybe rocks, roots, and worms at first—but this story suggests that the divine feminine is there too.

A plow creates order in a field: it makes straight furrows to house and protect the seeds, much as a mantra creates patterns in your mind and protects your thoughts. You must control the pressure, speed, and direction of the plow, much as a meditator controls the speed and direction of thoughts and breath.

A story of the Buddha's childhood says that he received his first insights into meditation by watching a farmer plow. The sight of the plow's tip meeting the earth, not too deep, not too shallow, and the long, smooth unfolding of each furrow, each one a match for the one before and the one after it, created a sense of deep calm and alert attention in the young Gautama. Just as regular meditation calls forth jewels of insight from the mind and brings us closer to our real nature, the plow creates deep, long, smooth, even channels in the earth—and may even reveal hidden treasure.

How has your practice helped you discover which gifts lie under the surface of your body and mind?

Do you meditate with a mantra? How does it help you weed out certain thought patterns and cultivate others?

How does this pose foster persistence and concentration over a long, sustained period of time (*Yoga Sutra* 1:14)?

To unearth the hidden treasures in your body and mind, you have to do your own practice—not someone else's, even if their practice seems preferable (*Bhagavad Gita* 18:47). Do you need to modify this pose to discover its benefits?

Rama draws his bow.

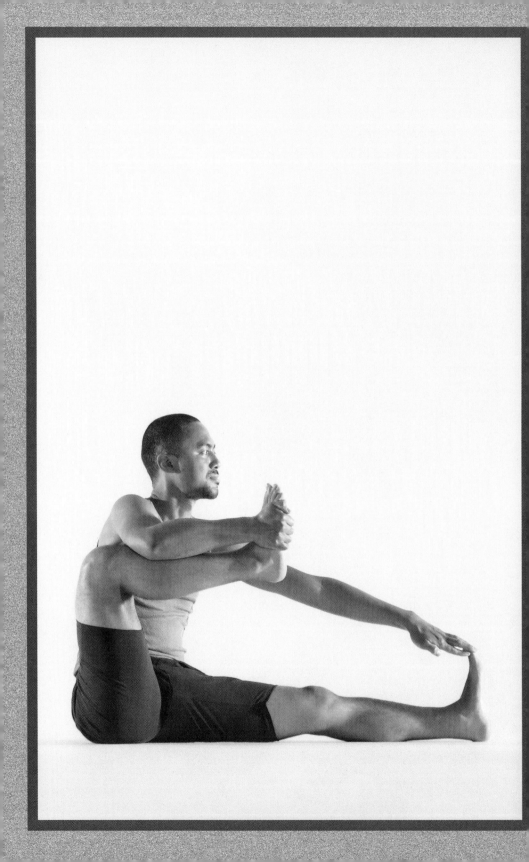

Sita Chooses Her Husband
Shooting Bow Pose / Akarna Dhanurasana

When Sita grew up, her father began planning for her marriage. In those days it was customary for the children of kings to marry partners selected to assure harmony among the people of their kingdoms. If the children were fortunate, they would grow to love their partners; if not, they would still have pleased their families and communities.

It so happened that King Janaka was the custodian of Lord Shiva's celestial bow. This bow was so heavy and so powerful that no mortal could lift it—except for, as Janaka discovered, his little daughter Sita. One day, the ball she was playing with rolled behind Shiva's bow. Astonished, Janaka watched his tiny scrap of a girl-child lightly move the enormous celestial bow out of her way to retrieve her toy. That gave him an idea. When Sita was old enough to choose a husband, Janaka decided to hold an archery contest for her *svayamvara*, the process by which a princess of marriageable age selects a husband from a list of candidates (*svayam* means "self" in Sanskrit, and *vara* means "groom").

Sage Vishvamitra, who knew that Rama and Sita were destined for each other, arranged for Rama and his brothers to attend Janaka's festival. As they entered the gates, Rama saw a young girl looking out of an upper window. Their gazes met. In that instant their hearts were joined forever, as indeed they had been since the beginning of time.

Scores of kings and warriors attended. No contestant could even move the bow, much less string it—except for Rama. At Vishvamitra's urging, Rama effortlessly raised the bow, strung it—and drew the string with such force that he shattered the shaft with a thunderous noise that shook the earth. It was clear who had won the contest, but "Sita has the final decision," said Janaka. And so Sita chose Rama as her husband.

King Janaka's custodianship of Shiva's bow symbolizes Shiva passing on the practice of yoga to Janaka, who, as we have seen, was a sage as well as a king and a karma yogi. Janaka's daughter, Sita, demonstrates her own *shakti* (power) through her ability to handle Shiva's bow.

Rama, with his own bow, is a symbol of one who has realized the unity of individual and ultimate reality. His bow is a symbol of the *sadhana* (sustained practice) which makes it possible for everyone to reach that goal.

Shooting Bow Pose / *Akarna Dhanurasana*

Shooting bow pose's name—*akarna dhanurasana*—comes from the Sanskrit *a* (toward or near), *karna* (ear), and *dhanur* (bow). Instructions for this pose in the fifteenth-century text *Hatha Yoga Pradipika* begin: "Grasp both toes with the hands [left with left, right with right]; keep one leg straight and draw the other to the ear as you would the string of a bow." Simple as this sounds, many people find this pose quite challenging to their strength and their hip flexibility.

Preparation

Getting a Feel for the Pose

Before trying full akarna dhanurasana (shown in the photo), get a feel for it by working one leg at a time. To start, work only the lifted leg.

Begin in the staff pose (*dandasana*) with both legs straight in front of you. Flex both feet.

Lean forward, hinging at the hips, and catch the outer edge of your left foot with the left hand, keeping your right leg extended on the floor.

For now, keep your right hand on the floor near your right hip.

Bending your left knee, draw the left foot back toward you and lift that leg until the left shin is parallel to the floor.

Now lift your right hand off the floor and use it to support the inner left heel. Using the strength of your arms, slowly draw that knee back until it is just outside your left shoulder. Maintain a 90-degree angle in your knee, keeping the foot high.

Sustaining the Pose

Keep your spine erect. Press down your extended right leg, from the sit bone to the heel. Lift both sides of your ribs and broaden your collarbones.

Keeping your left shin parallel to the floor, exhale and pull the left knee back. Don't let it drift out to the side; press the outer edge of your foot into your left hand. Now, still holding the left foot and keeping the shin parallel to the floor, move your left foot forward. "Pump" your left leg several times, using your arms to draw the knee back and forward.

Finally, keep the lifted left leg stable, exhale, and see if you can draw the knee even farther back. Make the foot level with your ear.

Releasing the Pose

Hold for a few breaths, exhale, and release. Rest for several breaths. Repeat on the other side.

Full Pose

Embodying the Pose

In this pose you will hold your right big toe with your right hand and your left big toe with your left hand.

Sitting with both legs extended, lean forward and catch the big toes. Wrap the first two fingers and the thumb of each hand around its respective big toe. If you can't reach your toes or can reach them only by caving in your chest and rounding your shoulders, wrap a strap around the ball of each foot and hold the ends of the straps.

Hold your left toe firmly. Keep your legs hip-width apart. Press the entire length of your left leg into the floor.

Exhaling, bend your right knee and draw your right foot along the floor toward you. Place the sole of your right foot on the floor, level with or slightly above your left knee.

Exhaling and keeping your right knee bent, lift the right leg. Draw the right knee back. Lift your right foot toward your ear.

Sustaining the Pose

Turn your head toward your left foot; sight along your left arm, as if you were gazing at the gold center of a target. The left arm is your arrow; the right arm draws the bowstring back.

Keeping your focus forward, relax your eyes, your tongue, your forehead, the base of your skull. Breathe.

Releasing the Pose

On an exhalation, release the pose and repeat on the other side.

Reflection

In this story, Rama and Sita come together through their mastery of Shiva's bow, a symbol of yoga.

The *Mundaka Upanishad* (2.2.4) uses archery as a metaphor for spiritual practice. The mantra Om is the bow. The target is supreme reality, or Brahman. The seeker's own self is the arrow. The senses are the string. Pulling back the string (withdrawing the senses from the claims of the sense objects) represents meditation, the process of redirecting energy from external objects to the real goal. With repeated, devoted practice over time, the individual self becomes as one-pointed as an arrow in flight; through that energetic concentration, the seeker hits the target. This sharp focus leads to a state of union between the individual soul and cosmic consciousness, or God. This is the state of yoga.

Shooting bow pose, akarna dhanurasana, puts us in touch with our tendency to strive. It is challenging, no doubt about it, but do you make it more effortful than it needs to be by gripping your jaw, your eyes, your breath? As you explore this pose, find the minimum of effort needed to achieve and hold it. When you get tired, which may happen fairly quickly, are you content to release the pose, or do you want to cling on, white-knuckled? *Sthira sukham asanam*, Patanjali tells us: "Asana is steady and comfortable." How does it feel to draw on your full strength and flexibility while maintaining ease? What limits you in this pose—is it arm strength, hip flexibility, something to do with your spine? What actions would you need to take (or avoid) to feel at home in akarna dhanurasana?

In practicing this pose, what is your goal? Is it to get your foot level with your ear while keeping your back straight? To maintain a calm focus while challenging your sense of balance and flexibility? What is at stake for you in your overall practice? Do considerations about physical performance distract you from the ultimate goal of spiritual union? Let this pose teach you how to be fully engaged physically while maintaining a meditative focus.

Although this pose involves strength, flexibility, and focus, it has its playful side too. In fact, the action of the legs is very much like a seated happy baby pose (*ananda balasana*), which you may enjoy as a preparatory practice for shooting bow pose.

Beginners: Don't be afraid to fall over the first time or two! Don't apologize for using your strap to lengthen your arm either. Remember little baby goddess Sita, who didn't let that big imposing bow get in the way of her play, and approach your practice with confidence and joy.

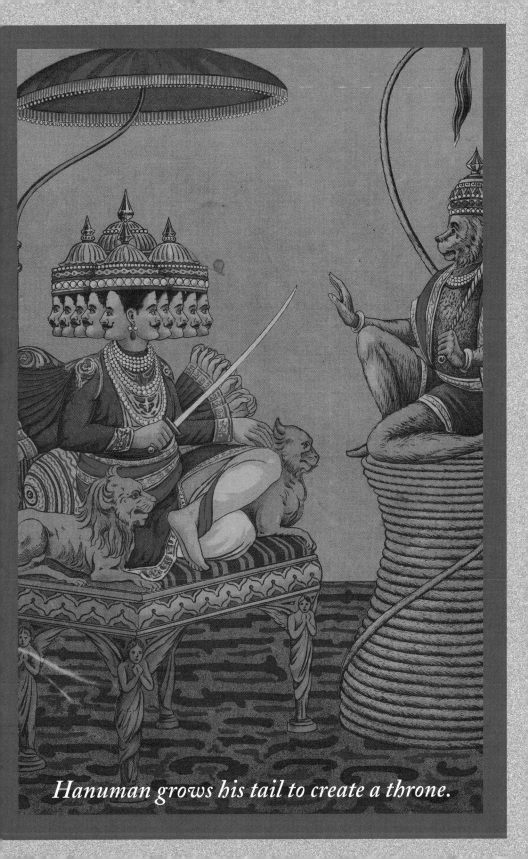

Hanuman grows his tail to create a throne.

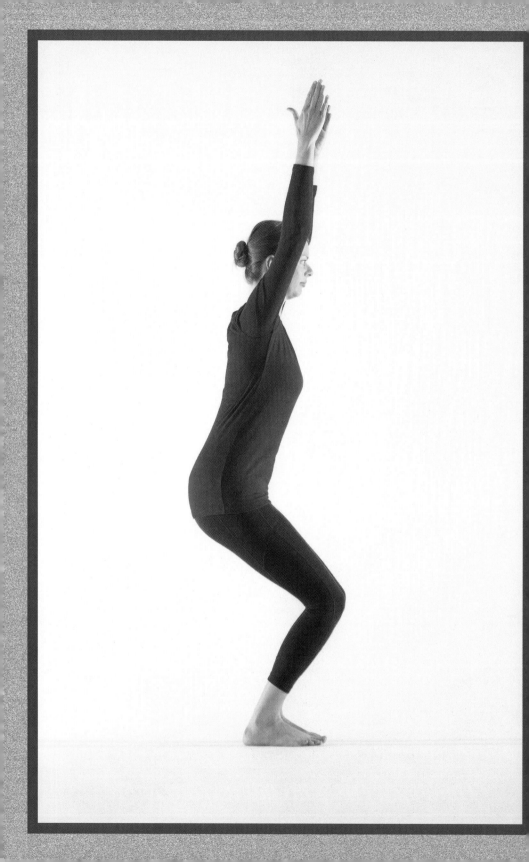

Rama Leaves His Throne and Hanuman Creates a Throne
Fierce Pose (Chair Pose) / Utkatasana

Soon after Rama's wedding, King Dasharatha's thoughts turned seriously to retirement. Rama was the eldest son and the best loved of all the four brothers. Everyone expected him to become king after Dasharatha, and everyone, including his brothers, rejoiced in the prospect. Why wait? Why not abdicate the throne and let Rama begin his life as *dharma raja*, a king who upholds righteousness, now?

Dasharatha consulted his advisers. They all applauded this decision and immediately began arranging the details of Rama's coronation, to be held the next morning at sunrise. When Rama himself was informed, he folded his hands and bowed to touch his father's feet. The news spread quickly throughout the palace. Rama's mother, Kaushalya, the senior queen, shared her joy by sending beautiful presents to her co-wives, Kaikeyi and Sumitra, and to the other women of the palace. They, too, were delighted.

But there was one person who was not delighted—Manthara, Kaikeyi's hunchback confidante. Manthara had a badly twisted spine, perhaps what we would now call scoliosis. She had borne a grudge against Rama from the time when, as a child, he had shot her painfully in the back with his toy bow and arrow. Her ill will now changed the expected course of events: Manthara prevailed upon her mistress to demand that Bharata sit on the throne and Rama go into exile.

The story of Rama and Sita's exile unfolds from this inauspicious beginning. Bharata, however, absolutely refused to be crowned king of Ayodhya. The most he would agree to was the role of acting regent in Rama's absence. To emphasize the point that his brother, not he, was the rightful ruler, he placed a pair of Rama's sandals on the throne as a symbol of the presence of their absent owner.

A throne is far more than an imposing piece of furniture; symbolically, it conveys power and authority to the one who sits on it. It places that one in a position to order other people's actions and lives. The ruler's decisions affect everyone in the kingdom. The person who occupies that throne, then, had better be wise, just, and prepared to let go of his own personal desires in the interest of the common good. First and foremost, he or she must be a dharma raja, both a servant of the people and an upholder of divine order. This is a huge responsibility. Everyone in Ayodhya expected Rama to be the next king, and everyone, except Manthara with her distorted thinking, knew that he was the best possible successor to Dasharatha.

Indian philosophy recognizes a special category of absence known as *pradvasambhava*, the absence of something or someone who was here, should be here, but no longer is. (For example, there was a cup on your desk when you left the room. When you came back, you noticed immediately that there was no cup. It should have been where you left it, but it was gone.) When Bharata placed Rama's sandals on the throne instead of sitting on it himself, he dramatized the absence of the ruler who ought to be occupying that throne. Rama's sandals told the people that the real ruler, the one who should be here, is not present.

Fierce Pose (Chair Pose) / *Utkatasana*

Utkatasana originates from the Sanskrit *utkata*, "fierce, proud, high, haughty, superior, immense, difficult"—all possible descriptors for the job of kingship! The pose is often called chair pose in English, because it looks as if you are sitting in an invisible chair, but this is no easy chair; it's more like a throne. Along with the full pose (shown in the photo), I have included a version practiced against the wall for support and for building strength.

Full Pose

Embodying the Pose

Stand straight, with your feet aligned, slightly wider than your hips.

Inhaling, lift your arms alongside your ears. Lengthen the arms from the shoulder blades; keep the fingers long and loose. (If you cannot raise your arms, bring the heels of your hands to the very tops of the thighs and press down; lift your spine and rib cage. Keep your shoulders down.)

Exhaling, bend your knees and fold at the hip crease, taking your hips back. Your bent knees will extend beyond your ankles.

Sustaining the Pose

Keeping your knees bent, sink a little deeper into the pose. Draw your navel back and up.

Keeping the back of the neck long, shoulders down, lift the base of the skull and the crown of the head—as if you were wearing a crown.

Find the tension, the balance, between working your legs powerfully, with stability, and lifting the arms and the crown of the head.

Where is the ease, where is the poise, in this pose? Notice your breath, and soften around the eyes.

Find the place where you lift and ground equally, energetically. The one on the throne must be grounded, in touch with the land and the people, but must also aspire upward, toward a higher power.

Are you ready to sit on this throne?

Releasing the Pose

Exhale, and lower the arms. Straighten the knees and hips.

Refinement

You can fine-tune the leg action in this pose by squeezing a block between your legs, above the knees; by taking your hands to the outer thighs, just above the knees, and creating resistance by pressing the thighs out and the hands in; or by practicing against a wall.

Variation Against the Wall

Embodying the Pose

Stand with the backs of your heels against the baseboard, about hip-width apart.

Keep your buttocks on the wall as you align your feet parallel to one another, about one foot-length from the wall. Bend your knees.

Are your knees ahead of your ankles? If so, step farther away from the wall until your knees are over your ankles. Keep your buttocks on the wall. Keep the feet parallel.

Now you can lift your arms overhead and take the navel back and up. Or press the heels of the hands into the tops of the thighs and take your navel back and up.

Pressing the feet into the floor, press your buttocks into the wall. Use the traction between the wall and your buttocks to slide the back of your pelvis down the wall.

Releasing the Pose

Exhale, and lower the arms. Straighten the knees and hips, step away from the wall, and come into mountain pose (*tadasana*).

Stay centered and breathe for a moment or two.

Reflection

In this story, there is confusion about who will occupy the throne, which represents leadership and authority. When Bharata places Rama's sandals on the throne, he is saying, "I will do what I can do, but the real power and authority of this office are not mine."

Have you ever been in a position to assume responsibility greater than you felt competent to handle? Like Bharata, you may have been called upon to take a job that you believed would be better filled by someone else—and yet, you were the one to do it.

How did that feel? Did it help, or might it help, to invoke the aid of some transpersonal authority?

Think about some of the other characters in this story; how do they reflect parts of your personality?

Manthara. I think we all have an inner "hunchback," some part of us that is small and twisted as a result of trauma or for reasons we don't even recognize—but there she is, fearful, resentful, vengeful, but convincing. Can you remember a time you let her take charge of your actions? How did that work out?

Kaikeyi. She has earned the king's gratitude and love without ever feeling the need to cash in on them. She is not jealous of Rama, whom she loves like her own son, until Manthara goes to work on her. What clouds her judgment? Is it a sense of misplaced loyalty? An ego-based attachment to Bharata? Why does she listen to her servant?

Dasharatha. This king, in his youth, was a renowned demon fighter. In an age when warriors fought from horse-drawn chariots, he earned the nickname Dasharatha, "ten chariots," because he could wreak as much damage on the battlefield as ten men. Under his rule, Ayodhya is peaceful and prosperous, and the old warrior wants only to leave rulership to his best-suited son. His old promise to Kaikeyi creates consequences he never foresaw, but his code forces him to honor it. Think: What must it be like for Dasharatha to be defeated by his own word? Have you made commitments which later proved difficult to live with? Is there an aspect of you that remains unreasonably loyal to old friendships or promises?

Rama. Representing the ideal man, Rama responds immediately and graciously to what must surely be an enormous disappointment—or, at least, a major shift in the course of events. He expects to become king in the morning—but no. Instead, he is exiled to the forest for fourteen years, because his stepmother, who has always seemed to love him, has gotten some crazy idea that her son should rule. Does Rama blame her or anyone else? Does he assert his rights? He does not. He accepts his father's edict, wrong though it is (and wrong though they both know it is), and prepares to go. Can you identify with Rama in having a goal snatched away when it was nearly achieved? How did you respond? What would it be like to be the kind of person who accepts what comes with complete equanimity?

Hanuman Creates a Throne

Another "throne" story from the *Ramayana* involves Hanuman. In his quest to rescue Sita, Hanuman flies to Lanka, where he is captured and brought before Ravana. Ravana, the very incarnation of pride and ego, ascends his impressively high throne and gazes contemptuously down on Hanuman. Hanuman, ever resourceful, uses his magical powers to make his tail grow . . . and grow . . . and grow, until its coils form a "throne" even higher than Ravana's, before bursting his bonds and flying away.

Reflection

In this story, a villain tries to exert power over a hero, but he is thwarted by the hero's ability to draw on his own superpowers and inner resources.

Have you ever been "looked down on"? Have you ever felt that someone was trying to elevate himself by demeaning you? How did you respond? What helped you tap into your inner resources?

Bharata refuses a throne that he knows not to be his. Hanuman creates a throne that elevates him, Rama's servant, above Ravana.

Hanuman's power and confidence are rooted in the knowledge that he is the servant and messenger of Rama. His faith in his Lord gives him confidence in himself, just as Bharata's faith allows him to govern in Rama's absence. Remember a time when you drew confidence from your place in a venerable lineage and did your best to behave in ways that honored that lineage and teacher.

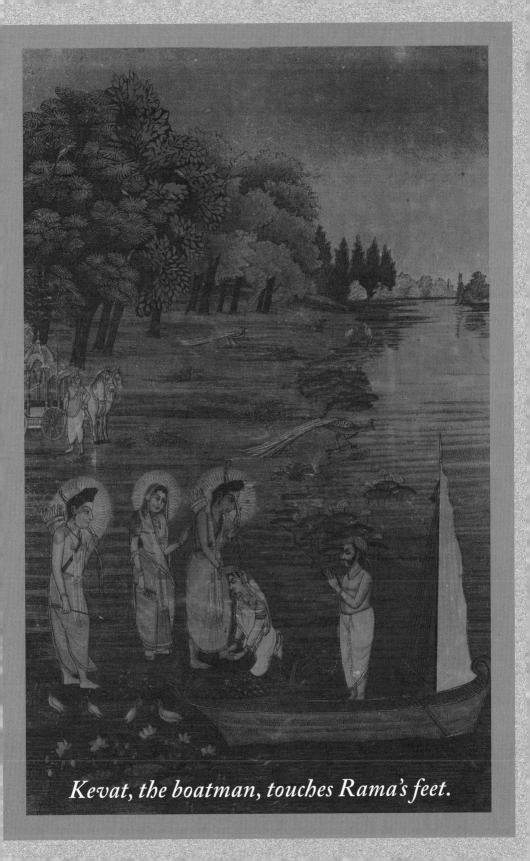

Kevat, the boatman, touches Rama's feet.

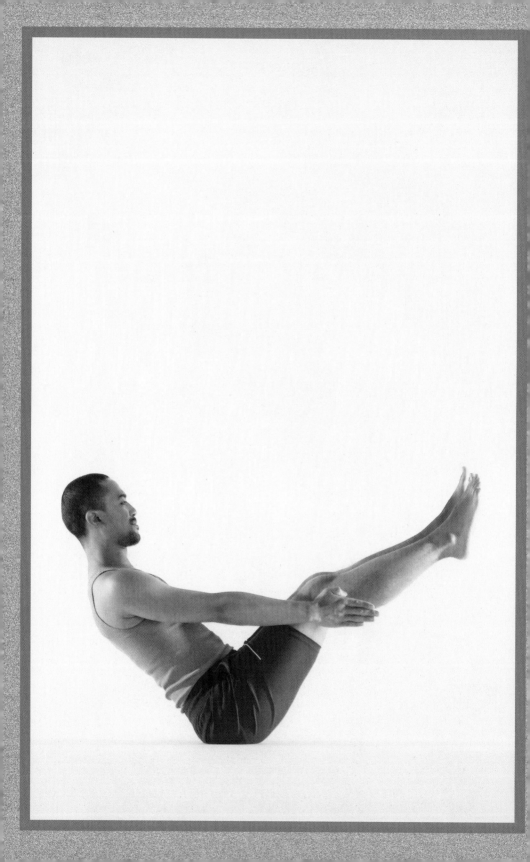

Crossing the River
Boat Pose / Navasana

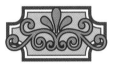

When Rama, Sita, and Lakshmana walked away from Ayodhya, the entire population followed them. In the evening Rama addressed the crowd. "You must go back," he said. "I am charged to stay away from Ayodhya for fourteen years, and I can hardly bring Ayodhya with me! Please go home now. Show your love for me by being kind to each other, supporting Bharata, and waiting peacefully for my return. Even if some of you never see me again in this life, know that I am with you in your hearts. You are mine and I am yours. But once we reach the river's edge, you cannot follow." He folded his hands, like lotus buds, raised them to his forehead, and bowed his head to the people.

Now, India is a land of rivers, and where there are rivers, there will inevitably be boats and *tirthas* (crossing places) to assist travelers on their journeys. Tirthas are often holy places associated with a deity or saint. Indian literature is rich with imagery involving boats and crossing water. Poets envision life in *samsara* (the world of senses and illusion) as the journey of a small craft across turbulent water, with God or one's spiritual practice as the skillful navigator who ferries us safely across.

When Rama, Sita, and Lakshmana left the people of Ayodhya behind, they had nearly reached the banks of the Ganga, the great mother of all rivers. There they sought a tirtha. Soon they saw a ferryman waiting by the shore with his small open boat, gazing peacefully at the water.

"Hey, Kevat!" they called. "Will you take us across?"

Kevat (the name simply means "boatman") looked up sharply. "Who's asking?" he questioned.

"Rama and Lakshmana, formerly of Ayodhya; and this is the lady Sita."

"Rama," said Kevat slowly, "I've heard your name. The touch of your foot turned a stone into a woman. What if you step into my boat and it turns into something else? No, Lord, sorry, I can't risk it."

Rama knew what Kevat meant about the touch of the Lord's foot. Once, on a journey, Rama had encountered Ahalya, turned to stone by her jealous husband, Sage Gautama, and restored to warm life by the touch of Rama's foot. Clearly, that story had spread.

After prolonged negotiations, Kevat agreed to carry the three wanderers to the other side of the river—but only if Rama would permit him to wash the dust from his feet and bow down to them. (In truth, this was what he had wanted all along; all that about being afraid his boat might turn into something else was just a ploy to be allowed to touch Rama's feet.)

On the other side, Sita offered her ring in payment. "By no means," said Kevat. "Lord, you, too, are a boatman. We are in the same line of work. I carry people across the river, but you carry them across the ocean of samsara—the world and all its problems. Your name alone is enough to assure safe passage!"

Once more, Rama allowed Kevat to touch his feet. "Brother," he said, "as you ferried me across the river, one day, I promise, I will free you from illusion."

In this story and the Ahalya story within it, we see the symbolic importance of the Lord's feet. They are the point at which the divine energy connects with the earth, providing a link—the human body—between earth and heaven. The touch of Rama's feet liberates Ahalya and transforms her from her "stuck" state, while Kevat, intuiting the power of those feet, wishes only to wash them and place his forehead on them. In India it is common practice to show respect by touching the feet of a revered elder, such as a parent or a teacher, and the feet of a spiritual leader are objects of veneration. According to Meher Baba:

> Spiritually the feet of the Master are above everything in the universe, which is like dust to them. When people come to a Perfect Master and touch his feet with their hands, they lay the burden of their *samskaras* [karmic impressions] on him. He collects the samskaras from all over the universe, just as an ordinary person, in walking, collects dust on his feet. There is a hoary custom that after the aspirant has the *darshana* [view or sight] of a Master and falls at his feet, he washes the Master's feet with milk and honey and places a coconut near them as his offering. Honey represents red samskaras, milk represents white samskaras, and the coconut represents the mind. Thus this convention, which has become established in some areas in connection with greeting the Masters, really symbolizes throwing the burden of all samskaras on the Master and surrendering the mind to him. Adoption of this inner attitude constitutes the most critical and important step which the aspirant must take in order to get initiated on the Path.
>
> (*Discourses*, Vol. 2, p. 94)

You might even say that the feet of a real master are both a tirtha and a boat—a place that eases our passage from our ordinary state of confusion and entanglement to the spiritual realm, and the vehicle that takes us across.

Boat Pose / *Navasana*

In *navasana*, your body mimics the shape of a small boat with a sail and oars. I like to introduce it in two stages: the full version (*paripurna*)—shown in the photo—and the half version (*ardha*). Both poses are powerful abdominal strengtheners! They challenge and strengthen the back and the abdominal muscles. The first pose resembles a *dhow*, a traditional Indian boat with a mast and a high, nearly triangular sail. The second is more like a rowboat or a canoe.

Full Boat Pose / *Paripurna Navasana*

This intermediate pose requires strength and concentration. Be sure you are engaging your abdominal muscles and not relying too much on your legs and hip flexors.

Embodying the Pose

Sit on your mat, on the front edge of your sit bones, with your knees bent and the soles of the feet on the floor. Hold your shins just below the knees. Lift your chest.

Lift your toes and begin to shift your weight back, lifting your chest, while lengthening your back.

Lift your heels, balance on your sit bones, and keep lifting your chest with a straight back.

Modifications

For people with low-back issues, a bent-knee or supported paripurna navasana is probably better. It can be done with the soles of the feet on the wall to help with balance or to provide support when the back and/or legs are weak. Another modification is to hold the backs of the thighs with your hands until you can extend the arms and legs. If you find this pose too difficult, ask a creative teacher for other suggestions.

Sustaining the Pose

Draw your shins parallel to the floor, and reach the arms straight forward. Your arms are the oars.

Draw your shoulder blades forward, plug the tops of the upper arm bones into the backs of the shoulder sockets, and extend your fingers.

Draw your navel strongly back and up.

On an exhalation, straighten the legs, lifting the feet to or above eye level. Keep drawing the navel back and up. Stay for a few breaths. Your spine is the mast, your legs are the sail.

Releasing the Pose

Bend the knees and place the feet back on the floor. Relax and breathe.

Half Boat Pose / *Ardha Navasana*

Embodying the Pose

Balance on your sit bones with your legs and arms extended in full boat pose.

After a few breaths, bend your elbows and place your fingers at the base of your skull (to support your neck), with elbows opening wide. Exhaling, squeeze your legs together and lower your legs halfway to the floor (or as close as you can without arching your low back).

Inhaling, lift your legs and raise your chest, reach your arms forward, and balance again in full boat. Remember to breathe.

Releasing the Pose

Bend your knees and lower your body to the mat. Relax.

Reflection

In this story, someone comes to a crossing point in their journey. To continue, they need assistance and a steady vehicle. The story draws a parallel between physically crossing the water and overcoming illusion.

What helps carry you "to the other side" of this pose? You begin with the feet on the floor—on the riverbank, as it were—and end in the same way. In between, your body lifts, it may sway, and you need to guide it. Observe your breath throughout. Can you keep it steady and your gaze calm even if the journey gets rough at times? Notice your eyes. Are they tense with effort? Can you keep them soft, perhaps focused on the tips of your big toes? As an experiment, try mentally repeating "Rama" as you hold the pose. Does it help to sustain you?

Think about your life as a voyage. Where have you encountered rough water, rocks, obstacles? Did you have a yoga practice then? What has helped keep you afloat through difficult times? Who or what has been a tirtha for you, helping you to cross over your difficulties?

Kevat tells Rama that they are colleagues: one carries travelers across the river, the other carries seekers across the waters of the illusory world to safe haven in the eternal. Indian philosophy is rich with references to multiple levels of reality. How does it transform your experience to think of your daily activities in symbolic terms?

Rama, Sita, and Lakshmana arrive at Sage Bharadvaja's ashram.

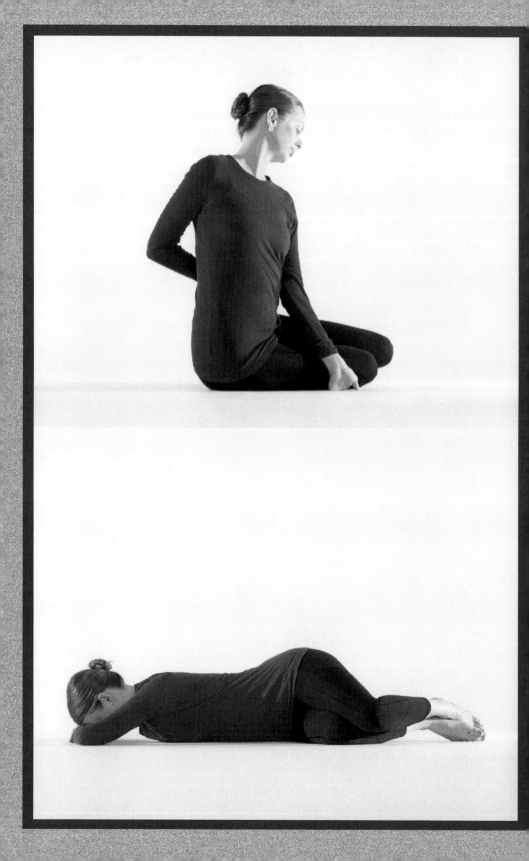

The Sage Who Waited for Rama

Sage Twist / Bharadvajasana

After Rama, Sita, and Lakshmana crossed the Ganga, to begin life as wandering renunciates, they sought refuge with the forest-dwelling yogis. (After all, Rama had been born to save the yogis' practices from the demons' depredations.) They traveled first to the ashram of the great sage Bharadvaja, whose name is familiar to yoga students from the asanas called after him and whose ashram still exists at Allahabad. As the three exiles approached his compound, Bharadvaja was preparing to perform the daily rituals of *arghya* and *padya*, washing the hands and feet of one's chosen deity.

On the outskirts of the ashram, Rama hailed a student: "Please tell your honored teacher that Rama, son of Dasharatha, is waiting at the forest's edge for permission to enter."

The excited student ran inside. "Master, someone who looks like a divinity has come! He says he is Rama."

With the offering ingredients still in his hands, Bharadvaja hastened to greet his guests. "Lord," he exclaimed, "I have been practicing austerities all these years in the hope of seeing the Self, and now you have come! You are Paramatman in human form, the highest of the high, the—I don't even know what to call you! All I know is that I am blessed and so happy to meet you, Rama—my Lord, my Lord!" And he fell at Rama's feet, dropping his ritual implements in his excitement.

"Get up, Bharadvaja," said Rama kindly. He helped the older man to stand, and he embraced him. "You are a sage, and we are only wanderers in the forest, rulers without a kingdom. Please give us shelter in your ashram; let us rest and refresh ourselves before we continue on our journey."

"Of course, Lord! You and your companions are welcome to stay here as long as you like."

Looking at the water and vessels that Bharadvaja had dropped in his eagerness to greet them, Rama smiled and gestured toward them. "I apologize; we interrupted your practice. May we participate now?"

And Bharadvaja, who every day washed the feet and hands of the Supreme Lord in his imagination, now washed the dusty, brown, muscular feet of that very Lord in human form. And he was supremely happy.

Sage Twist / *Bharadvajasana*

There are several poses named for Sage Bharadvaja. This family of poses are all twists, some simple, some requiring considerable flexibility. I have selected one simple seated pose (shown in the upper photo) and one reclining pose with two variations: a reclining variation without a bolster (shown in the lower photo) and one with a bolster (described below) for those who may require or prefer the ease it provides.

Seated Bharadvajasana

Embodying the Pose

Sit on the floor, with the legs stretched straight out in front, as in staff pose (*dandasana*).

Exhaling, lean on your right hand, bend the knees, and slide your legs along the floor until the sides of both feet rest on the floor beside your left hip.

Reach the left sit bone toward the floor; your weight will be more on the right hip.

Exhaling, turn your navel and trunk to the right. Draw your left arm across the thighs, and slip your left fingers or hand under the right knee, with the palm facing down. (If you have trouble getting the left hand under your knee, place the back of the left hand outside the right knee, palm facing outward.)

Lift your right arm to shoulder height. Exhaling, draw your right arm behind your back, with the palm facing outward, thumb pointing upward. If possible, hold your upper left arm with your right hand. (Alternately, take the right arm behind your back, closer to the floor, as close to the left hip as possible; press the fingers into the floor, and lift your chest.)

Exhaling, turn your head to the left and gaze over your left shoulder. Stay for several breaths, up to a minute.

Sustaining the Pose

Picture your spine as a washcloth held by two huge, benevolent hands. The stress and exhaustion in your body are the soapy water in the washcloth. As you exhale in this pose, imagine wringing the washcloth of your spine to rid it of soapy water (stress); as you inhale, imagine rinsing the washcloth with clean, fresh water.

Releasing the Pose

Exhaling, slowly untwist, and return to dandasana for a few relaxed breaths. Repeat on the other side.

Reclining (Supta) Bharadvajasana with Bolster

Embodying the Pose

Sit on the floor, legs extended. Place a bolster at a right angle to your left hip. Exhaling, bend the knees and bring your bent legs to rest by your right hip.

Take your left hand to the midline of the bolster. Exhaling, slide your arm down the midline of the bolster, lengthening your spine and opening the spaces between your lower ribs. You will be nearly lying on your side on the bolster. Take your left hand to the floor under your left shoulder, keeping your body low. Take your right hand to the floor under your right shoulder. Now, press into both hands and lift your torso.

Exhaling, press more into the left hand, and turn your navel toward the bolster. Bend your elbows and slip both forearms under the bolster, palms up, as if you were hugging the bolster to your chest. Turn your head to look over your left shoulder (away from your knees). If this strains your neck, then keep the head facing in the direction of your knees.

Sustaining the Pose

Check the relationship of your shoulders to your ears. If the shoulders are up near your ears, add more height: place an additional blanket on top of the full length of the bolster, and lie down again; your upper arm bones will now be at nearly a right angle to the floor, creating space between the shoulder and the ear. Be high enough that you don't feel propped up on your elbows; let the elbows rest very lightly on the floor. The height of your props is a matter of your body's proportions; people with long upper arm bones will need more height than people with shorter upper arm bones.

Once you have established the correct support, release your body into the pose. Inhale and exhale through the nose, visualizing the inbreath moving down your spine to the tailbone and the exhalation moving up the spine and out the crown of the head.

Releasing the Pose

Exhaling, slowly untwist, and return to dandasana for a few relaxed breaths. Repeat on the other side.

Reflection

In this story, a dedicated yogi spends years in practice, visualizing an encounter with the Divine. Unexpectedly, his patience bears fruit, and practice succeeds beyond his wildest expectations.

Bharadvaja visualizes washing Rama's feet and hands every day as part of his devotions. He pictures it in detail, with devotion, every day, for a long time. Then, in his old age, the object of his devotion manifests.

This is exactly how the *Yoga Sutra* tells us we should practice. In *Yoga Sutra* 1:13, Patanjali speaks of practice (*abhyasa*) as choosing actions that lead to a stable, tranquil state (*stithau*), and in 1:14, of doing those actions for a long time, without a break, and with sincere devotion.

Although there are simple versions of this sage twist, it may take a long time and much patience to master the full pose. You can't force yourself into a deep, complex twist without risking injury. Once you are in a twist, stay there and breathe; don't just pop in and out. Maybe when you first encountered bharadvajasana you thought there was no way your body would ever inhabit this pose comfortably. As you stay with it, though, you find your patience rewarded with a deep, easy, stable posture.

You may not have a devotional practice like Bharadvaja's, but visualization can be a powerful ally in your asana practice. Let's say you are afraid to kick up into a full arm balance. You want to do it, you understand the principles, but your body simply will not cooperate. Mentally, you rehearse the movements you want to do, imagining the muscles involved, how you will breathe, how it will feel when both feet sail up and touch the wall. Picture this every day, in detail, patiently, without pressure. One day, when you approach the pose, your body will realize, "We know how to do this!" and up it will go.

Think of a time when you pictured something you longed for but didn't necessarily expect ever to receive. Maybe it was a job, a home, a pet, your graduation ceremony. What happened? How would you feel to look up one day and see your heart's desire in front of you?

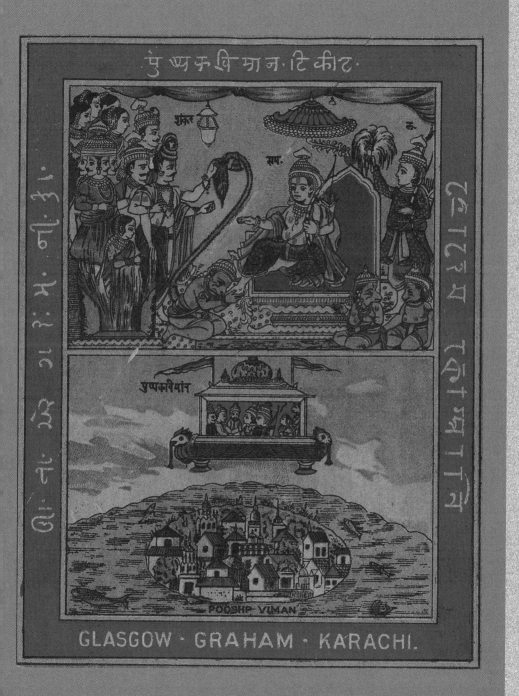

*A vimana, flying machine, soars above
the world.*

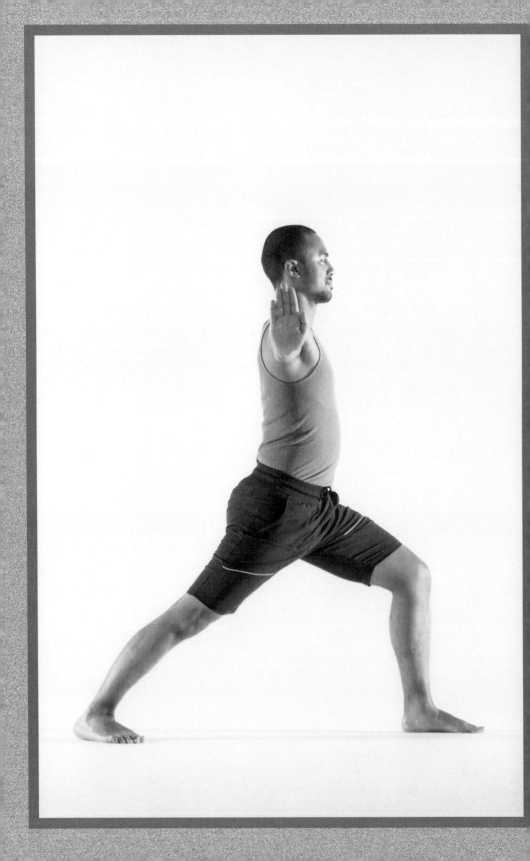

Sita's Abduction
Airplane Pose / Vimanasana

On their journey in exile, Rama, Sita, and Lakshmana took refuge in the Dandaka Forest, home to many hermits as well as a haunt of demons. On the bank of the Godavari River, they built a hermitage in a beautiful grove of five great banyan trees (*panch vati* in the local language). After subduing some of the demons harassing the local rishis, they lived there tranquilly, in the area we now know as Nasik.

One day, the *rakshasi* (demoness) Surpanakha, a sister of the demon king Ravana, caught sight of Rama and fell instantly in love. Disguising herself as a beautiful woman, she approached Rama and offered herself to him. Rama pointed out Sita, a short distance away, saying he was already married. Tactfully, he refused Surpanakha, telling her that a woman like her should not have to be a co-wife.

Resuming her own form, Surpanakha flew at poor Sita to tear her apart and remove this obstacle to her union with Rama. Lakshmana leapt to Sita's rescue, drawing his sword and swiping off Surpanakha's ears and nose. "I'd have cut off your ugly head," he said coldly, "but I don't kill women." The rakshasi fled, howling, to show Ravana her wounds and beg his help in avenging herself.

Ravana was unsympathetic. "You deserve it," he said, "offering yourself to a human!"

"But," said Surpanakha, who knew her brother's temperament, "you should see his wife! She is exquisite. In fact, she's worthy of your harem, Ravana. You should have her. Get her for your own, and leave those two men to me."

Ravana was intrigued. He got in touch with his uncle Maricha, one of the demons who harassed the local rishis by defiling their sacrificial altars with blood, flesh, bones, and filth. Maricha had already encountered Rama, so he tried to talk Ravana out of kidnapping Sita and battling Rama, warning that it would be the ruin of Ravana and Lanka. Ravana ordered Maricha, under penalty of death, to help him in his scheme. Maricha chose to die by Rama's bow rather than at the hand of Ravana.

Transforming himself into an enchanting golden deer with sapphire eyes, Maricha frolicked charmingly in the glade outside Rama and Sita's ashram. Sita was entranced: "Oh, the darling deer! Can't we have it as a pet?"

"I don't think that's a real deer," said her husband.

"But it's so sweet! Rama, please, please catch it for me."

Reluctantly, Rama hoisted his bow to go after the supposed deer, telling Sita not to leave the house and to obey Lakshmana's every instruction, and requesting Lakshmana not to leave Sita unattended.

When he came upon Maricha, he shot the demon through the heart. With his dying breath, Maricha shouted in a perfect mimicry of Rama's voice, "Lakshmana! Help me!"

Back at the hermitage, Lakshmana and Sita heard this cry. "Oh, go quickly and help him!" said Sita.

Lakshmana demurred, feeling more certain than ever that this was a trick. They argued. Finally Lakshmana drew a magic circle around the house, protected by mantras, and instructed Sita not to step outside that circle on any account until he returned with Rama.

Scarcely had he left when an elderly rishi in modest garments, holding a begging bowl, appeared. Standing shyly at the door, he asked for alms. This was Ravana. Although Sita had been warned not to step one toe outside the door, she was deceived by Ravana's mild disguise. She crossed the threshold and the supposed rishi seized her.

At first he tried to flatter Sita. He admitted that he was no ascetic, but a king, so smitten by her beauty that he had resorted to this ruse in order to be near her. He swore his love and offered her a prominent place in his harem. Sita, horrified, rejected his advances. Then Ravana bared his fangs, assumed his own horrific, ten-headed form, seized Sita in his twenty arms, hauled the screaming, struggling queen up into his *vimana* (flying chariot), and streaked like an evil meteor toward Lanka.

As they flew, Sita cried desperately to the trees, the birds, and the animals, "I am Sita, Rama's wife! Help me, brothers and sisters, children of my Mother Earth! Tell Rama! Mark my trail!" And, one by one, she flung pieces of her jewelry over the edge of the vimana to the earth.

The Indian epics refer, tantalizingly, to flying machines, vimanas, which flew of their own accord, like birds—multistoried constructions, unlike the classic horse-drawn chariots that carried warriors into battle and deities such as Surya, the sun, across the sky. The most famous of these flying machines was Pushpaka, a flowery vimana created for Kubera, the god of wealth, which Ravana had stolen.

Pushpaka is said to have been two stories high. Inside its elegant exterior were spacious, windowed rooms from which the occupants could view the scenery in comfort. As it passed like a bright cloud through the sky, Pushpaka made a musical sound. And it had a special feature—no matter how many passengers it carried, there was always a vacant seat.

Airplane Pose / *Vimanasana*

Airplane pose (*vimanasana*) imitates the shape of a flying machine. It resembles warrior 1 pose (*virabhadrasana 1*), but the arms are held parallel to the floor.

Embodying the Pose

Stand with your feet parallel and hip-width apart, your back toward the wall.

Take a long step forward with your left foot, and take your right foot back so that the back of your right heel is in contact with the baseboard.

Exhaling, bend your left knee. Look down; make sure your left shin is vertical.

Draw your left thighbone parallel to the floor so that the knee forms a right angle; less of an angle is fine if your hips are tight, but don't take the knee beyond your ankle.

Place your hands on your hips. Make your hips parallel to the wall by moving your right hip forward, away from the wall, and your left hip back, toward the wall.

Inhaling, lift your arms to shoulder height, fingers extended. Keeping your fingers extended, begin to raise the fingers as if you could form a right angle between them and your palms.

Now, with your palms facing out, press through the heels of both hands. Notice how this action "sets" the tops of the arm bones securely in your shoulder sockets. Now bring your hands back into line with your wrists and arms.

Sustaining the Pose

Inhale to the center of your sternum; exhaling, expand the space behind your heart—lengthen both arms from the inner edge of your shoulder blades to the tips of the fingers. Keep the arms parallel to the floor.

Release the top rim of your glutes down. Lengthen the tailbone toward the space between your feet. Ground your back heel into the baseboard.

Lift the crown of your head toward the ceiling. Keep the eyes and jaw soft.

Slide the skin over your breastbone up, over the tops of your shoulders and down the back, to the bottom tips of your shoulder blades. Widen the shoulder blades away from one another. Breathe calmly and smoothly. Feel the creative tension between the firm grounding of your back heel and the light, expansive feeling in your upper chest.

Releasing the Pose

To come out, lower the arms, straighten your front leg, and step your feet together. Repeat on the opposite side.

Finally, stand equally on both feet. Feel the solid earth under you.

Reflection

This story is about being deceived and carried away by illusion born from desire. Ravana is lost by it. But Sita regains her ground by being resourceful and by accepting help.

Since childhood, I've had flying dreams. In the dreams, I run with long strides and my arms outstretched until I press hard with my back heel, lift off the earth, and soar into the sky. I can control how high I go by raising or lowering my arms. I feel so happy and free!

When I got older and studied psychology, I learned that flying dreams can be a sign of an overactive nervous system. You may feel temporarily energetic, but beware: a crash awaits you! Too much lightness and motion, as in air travel, can be draining. Jungian psychology says that flying dreams show a desire to transcend your limitations, expand your consciousness; but they also indicate inflation, an exaggerated sense of self-importance. The downside to psychological inflation is that it is false, an attempt to compensate for unaddressed issues. Instead of solving problems, it takes you "above your self," into arrogance, inviting a fall.

This is exactly what happens to Ravana in this story. His lust for Sita carries him away. His inflated ego insists that he can overpower Sita, and her husband and anyone else who would restrain him.

Sita, in her own way, is captured by desire too. She wants the golden deer and insists that Rama catch it for her. And her desire to help the supposed mendicant overrides Rama and Lakshmana's instructions not to leave the hut. Following these desires, she loses her focus on Rama and "loses her ground" to Ravana.

Once Ravana seizes control, Sita cannot save herself, but she can and does call for help. She yells aloud that she has been taken, and strategically drops items that can identify her and her route. Notice, she throws her jewelry and identifying items to the earth. This is important; she does what she can to connect with the earth, to ground herself and assert her identity.

While the *Ramayana* and its events are widely accepted in India as historical, they are also a powerful teaching story. My teacher Sri Brahmananda said Sita represents mind or individual consciousness; Rama represents Ishvara, universal consciousness; and Ravana represents the obstacles to one-pointedness, or the ego, with his ten heads and twenty arms, symbolizing the claims of the senses. Individual consciousness and Ishvara should always be united. When ego, or desire for sense objects, takes over, the mind gets separated from Ishvara and is carried away in a fantasy, symbolized by Pushpaka, the luxury vehicle. Flying off in Pushpaka means letting your thoughts and ego run rampant: "I will do this, I will have that, I will be rich, successful, envied . . ." There is always room for one more seat in Pushpaka, just as there is no end to uncontrolled thoughts.

Patanjali's list of obstacles (*Yoga Sutra* 1:30–31) includes carelessness, inability to withdraw from sense cravings, confused understanding, and mental distractions. Which of these do you see at work in this story? In your story? Can you recall a time when you were swept off your feet, as it were, by a person, a train of thought, or a set of circumstances that appeared compelling, but proved to be false and dangerous—illusory? Has a "golden deer" appeared in your life, too beautiful to be real but too attractive to ignore? Do you ever catch yourself engaging in addictive thinking or behavior? Of course you do; we all do. What helps "bring you back to earth"?

Notice the wonderful expansive feeling of your arms and chest in the pose; it feels infinite! But stay too long, or lose the grounding in your legs, and your pose will falter.

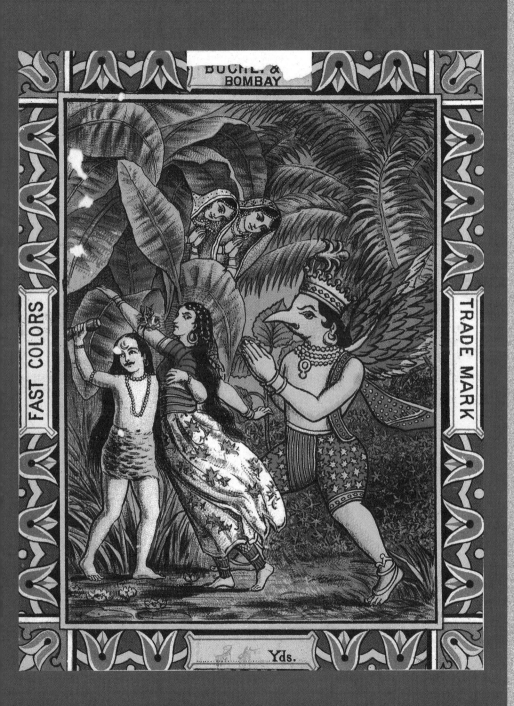

*Jatayu urges Ravana to free Sita,
before attacking him.*

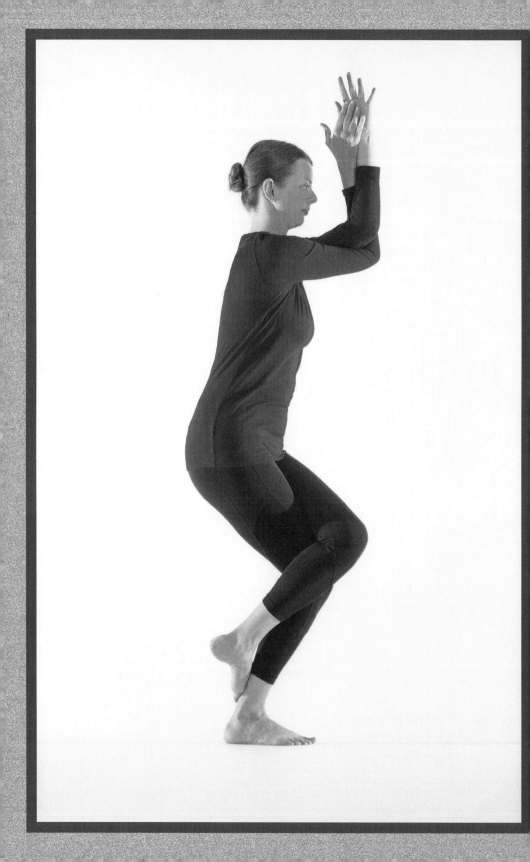

Jatayu Attempts to Rescue Sita

Eagle Pose / Garudasana

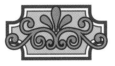

Although it is called eagle pose in English, *garudasana* is named for Garuda, described in South Asian tradition as a huge, mythical bird having the golden body of a man, an eagle's white face, and red wings. He is the king of the bird community, the enemy of snakes, the vehicle of Lord Vishnu, and the friend of humans. Jatayu, the nephew of Garuda, is sometimes referred to as a vulture in translations of the *Ramayana*, but he is neither a vulture nor an eagle in the usual sense—he is this huge, celestial, mythical bird.

Jatayu was an old friend of Rama's father, Dasharatha. In their youth they had served together to protect the rishis of the Dandaka Forest from raids by rakshasas.

When Ravana abducted Sita and carried her off to Lanka in Pushpaka, Jatayu was sitting contemplatively on a treetop, his keen eyes scanning the world's horizon. He remembered valiant exploits from his youth, battles and comrades won and lost. One incident above all haunted him. He had challenged his older brother, Sampati, in a race to the sun. Jatayu was winning, but in his rash young exuberance he flew so close to the sun that his wings began to smoke. Sampati flung himself between the sun and his brother, burning both his own wings so severely that he plummeted to earth and had to live the rest of his life as a wingless, flightless amputee. "That should have been me," brooded Jatayu.

Lost in memories of his brother, he heard Sita's screams. With his eagle-like gaze, he saw Ravana's chariot hurtling through the sky and flew into action. He hit the chariot head-on, knocking it to the ground. After trying, but failing, to convince Ravana to release Sita, Jatayu ferociously attacked him with his sharp beak, tearing claws, and powerful beating wings. But he was no match for the demon king's ten heads and twenty arms; for every head or limb that he lost, Ravana grew another before the first had finished falling. Jatayu fought fiercely, valiantly, and increasingly hopelessly. Finally Ravana hacked off both of Jatayu's wings and zoomed south toward Lanka, while Sita huddled in silent shock on the floor of the beautiful luxury chariot.

As Jatayu lay mortally wounded, Rama and Lakshmana arrived on foot, tracking Sita. With failing breath, the fallen warrior told them in broken phrases: "Sita, Ravana, headed south . . . Rama, please. I was your father's comrade. Kill me. It is a blessing to die at the Lord's hands and in his presence." Rama, always kind but never sentimental, shot one swift arrow through Jatayu's brave heart. Then he and Lakshmana gathered wood, built a pyre, and performed Jatayu's funeral rites with as much care as if they had been his sons.

Eagle Pose / *Garudasana*

There are many variations of *garudasana*. Some variations show the same leg and arm crossed on top while other variations call for alternating with the right arm crossed on top and the left leg crossed on top. We will do the version with the same arm and same leg crossed on top (shown in the photo).

Embodying the Pose

Begin in mountain pose (*tadasana*), standing with your feet parallel and hip-width apart, your arms at your sides, and the crown of your head lifted toward the ceiling. Widen your peripheral vision. Inhaling, raise the arms to shoulder level with palms facing up.

Exhaling, place the left arm over the right; stack the arms with the left elbow on top.

Bend the elbows. The backs of the forearms should now be parallel, with the backs of the hands facing one another.

Wrap your forearms around each other until the palms touch. Keep the wrists in line with your forearms and lengthen your fingers. (If you cannot join the palms without straining your wrists, keep the hands parallel with the backs facing each other.)

Press the forearms in opposite directions. Notice the stretch across your "wings" (shoulder blades).

Shift your weight to the right foot. Bend your knees. (If you cannot bear full weight on only one leg, do not wrap the legs; keep your feet parallel, bend the knees, and take your hips back into a high squat.)

Cross your left leg over the right leg, above the knee.

Place the left foot behind your right lower leg, and hook the left big toe or foot over the right calf or ankle. (Now, on both the top half of your body and the bottom half of your body, the left limb is on top of the right limb and wraps around the right limb.)

Sustaining the Pose

Balance. Draw your hip points toward one another. Draw your navel back and up. Widen your back lungs. Breathe.

Imagine yourself an eagle poised in the sky, still to all outward appearances but intensely active and present inwardly. Breathe smoothly.

Lift the base of the skull. Lean slightly forward from the hip crease, but lift your chest.

Widening through the back of the shoulder blades, press the forearms in opposite directions.

Focus your gaze on the inner edge of your hands, like an eagle soaring and sighting.

Pay attention to the qualities of softness or tightness in your breath, your body, and your eyes. Notice if your eyes want to tense and move forward, especially when you focus keenly on your hands. Can you be soft and focused at the same time? Can you keep your muscles active and your breath soft?

Experiment with breathing into your lower back lungs, expanding the ribs like wings on the inhalation. Breathe like a gliding bird.

Releasing the Pose

Remain in this pose for 30–60 seconds. Then return to tadasana. Breathe and relax. Repeat with the opposite arm and leg on top.

Reflection

In this story, the old warrior Jatayu sacrifices his life to aid Sita, and balances an old debt.

Garuda is the vehicle of Vishnu, the preserver, sustainer, and protector of creation (and Rama is one of Vishnu's incarnations). Vishnu's name comes from the root *vish*, "to enter into, to pervade." Vishnu sustains, preserves, and protects the universe by entering into it and never, for a moment, being absent—just as, in meditation, you choose an object of focus and then, to sustain your meditation, you continually choose that same object again and again. Think what it means to preserve and sustain. What qualities would you need to be the vehicle of the preserver? How do you breathe as the vehicle of preservation? How does that energy feel in your muscles and bones?

Take the pose again. As you sustain it, let your awareness pervade every part of your body, your breath, your sense organs. Be equally present everywhere. When you find any part of your attention wavering, renew your commitment to being present. Where is this most challenging?

Rama's enemy, Ravana, personifies egocentrism. When Ravana kidnaps Sita, his action disrupts creation, just as desires and claims of the ego arise to disrupt your practice. Like Garuda, Jatayu's natural state is one of sustained attention, and his dharma is selfless service: helping to protect creation and everything in it. He tries to fulfill his role but, valiant though Jatayu is, the ego is hydra-headed—cut off one head, and another pops right up. Ask yourself: When ego concerns disrupt my practice, how do I protect it?

Why does Rama kill Jatayu in this story? From compassion. It is, as Jatayu says, a blessing to die at the Lord's hands or in his presence. In Indian tradition, such a death virtually assures the devotee's liberation. Although this part of the story makes us feel sad, it also reminds us that, as Krishna says, it is better to perform one's own dharma, even if imperfectly, than to try to fulfill the dharma of another (*Bhagavad Gita* 18:47). Jatayu's dharma is to be a warrior. His one regret in life is that he put his brother in danger, with tragic results. Now, against great odds, he does his utmost, and though he fails to rescue Sita, the result for him is release from suffering, granted by the Lord himself. He loses the battle but wins the war. Think about this. Have you ever tried your best in a difficult situation and thought you'd failed, only to find that the end result was much, much better than you could have planned?

Jatayu has lived much of his life burdened by shame and regret for the injuries his brother incurred protecting him. This is sometimes called survivor guilt. It affects military veterans and others who survive a devastating, traumatic experience from which others do not survive or survive with a life-changing injury. When I worked as a chaplain in a Veterans Health Administration hospital, I met soldiers who were haunted most of all by the terrible things that had happened to their comrades. Perhaps Jatayu's "suicide mission" to rescue Sita is motivated in part by his wish to somehow repay Sampati. Perhaps, in sacrificing his wings for Sita, he balances his karmic debt to the brother who lost his own wings for Jatayu's sake.

Has anything in your life left you with a sense of survivor guilt? How has it affected your choices and actions?

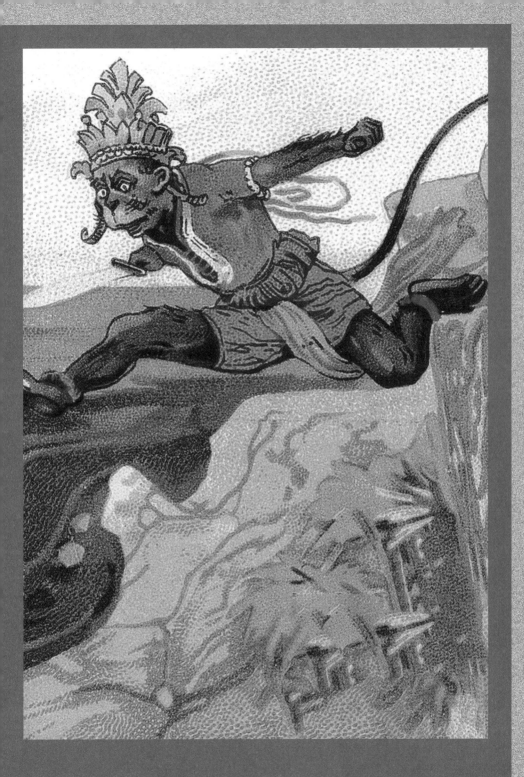

Hanuman leaps over the sea to the rescue.

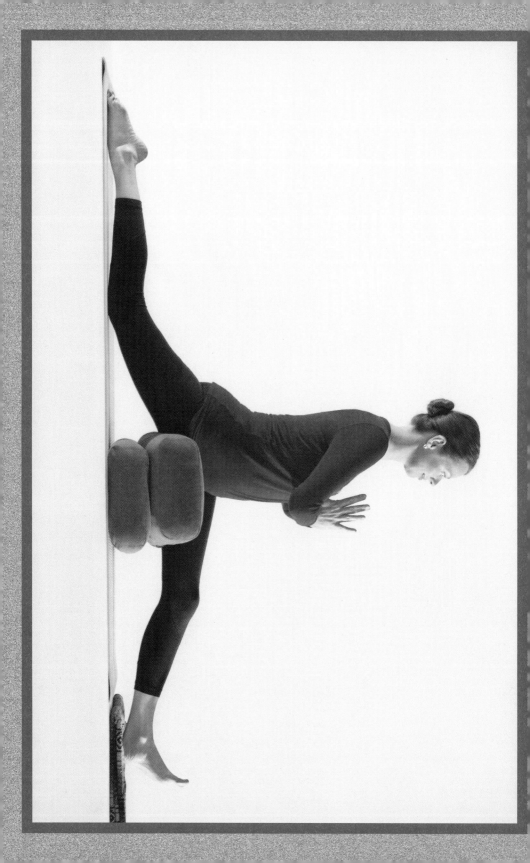

Hanuman's Leap
Monkey Pose / Hanumanasana

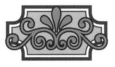

After performing Jatayu's funeral rites, Rama and Lakshmana walked south, searching for Sita's trail. After some time they encountered a band of Vanaras. Today we are not sure exactly who the Vanaras were. Some sources refer to them as monkeys, and the name of the pose known as *vanarasana* is often translated as "monkey pose." There is archaeological evidence for a tribal group of people living near Kishkinda (modern Hampi) as early as Neolithic times, who called themselves Vanaras and used a monkey as their totem. So it is possible that the original Vanaras were forest-dwelling, indigenous people whose tribal symbol was a monkey.

The king of this particular band of Vanaras was Sugriva. Sugriva and his people were in exile themselves, having lost their kingdom to Sugriva's brother Vaali, who had also taken Sugriva's wife. These Vanaras had seen Pushpaka speeding through the sky, heard a woman's screams, and retrieved some of the jewelry that Sita dropped. When

Rama and Lakshmana arrived on foot, the first person they met was Sugriva's minister, Hanuman. Hanuman introduced them to Sugriva, whose predicament was strikingly similar to Rama's. Sugriva offered to furnish an army in exchange for Rama's aid in resolving issues with Vaali. This task accomplished, Rama, Lakshmana, and Hanuman set out to rescue Sita, accompanied by an army of monkey people and their allies, the bears.

Hanuman's father was Vayu, the wind. His mother, Anjana, was a celestial nymph who took birth in the Vanara community precisely so that Hanuman could be born. The baby monkey came into the world endowed with supernatural strength, including the ability to fly and leap great distances. Throughout South Asia today, he is renowned for his physical strength, bravery, and devotion.

From Jatayu and the Vanaras, Rama learned that Sita had been taken to Ravana's capital, the island kingdom of Lanka. But where, precisely, on the island was she? And how would her rescuers span the distance across the sea to find her? Everyone looked at Hanuman, the only one who could both fly and leap vast distances.

Rama entrusted Hanuman with his ring to show to Sita as proof of his allegiance. Hanuman climbed to the top of a bluff facing the sea. Then, with a force that made the sand fly and the waves run backward, he stretched his mighty legs. The power of his back leg propelled him into the sky, while his front foot re-e-e-ached for the shore of Lanka. Hands clasped as in prayer, he held Rama's ring to his heart.

After searching the city and Ravana's palace, he found Sita sitting sadly in a grove of Ashoka trees patrolled by rakshasi guards. Flinging himself into a tree above her, he called softly, "Rama, Rama . . ." and dropped Rama's ring into her lap. Sita looked up, amazed, to see a little monkey that leapt playfully to her shoulder, chattering quickly: "Lady, don't worry! I come from Rama! It's his ring! I'm Hanuman! Don't worry, we'll rescue you! Take it! It's from Rama!" This seemed unusual, even to someone who had been kidnapped in a sky carriage by a shape-shifting demon. But Sita recognized her husband's ring, and although she had no idea who this monkey was, her heart told her to trust him when he assured her that Rama was coming with an army to rescue her.

Monkey Pose / *Hanumanasana*

This is a demanding pose. Most people find that they need regular practice, and quite possibly some support, before they can attain steadiness and ease in this pose. Remember Patanjali's words in *Yoga Sutra* 2:46: *Sthira sukham asanam*—"asana should be steady and comfortable." If the full pose seems too hard for you, try the modified variation (shown in the photo).

Full Pose

Embodying the Pose

Monkey pose (*hanumanasana*) is a full frontal split. If your hips, shoulders, and groin are very open, then kneel on the floor and place your palms down, under your shoulders.

Exhaling, press into your palms and lift your knees off the floor.

Stretch the left leg forward between your hands, and the right leg back.

Exhaling, press the legs and sit bones into the floor, and bear the weight through your arms and hands. The back of your left thigh should be on the floor, and the front of your right thigh (up to the groin, if possible) should be on the floor.

Press the top of your right foot and left heel into the floor and stretch the legs evenly.

Exhaling, bring your hands to *namaste* (*anjali mudra*, or prayer position) in front of your heart. Keep the hips level.

On the next exhalation, take your arms overhead, in line with your ears. Widen the shoulder blades and lift the inner collarbones. Stretch your outer collarbones toward your inner arms. Slide the rib cage toward your head. Keeping the elbows extended, join the hands overhead.

Sustaining the Pose

Imagine a tail extending from the base of your spine. Not all monkeys have long tails, but Hanuman does. Lengthen your tail, to the tip of the coccyx, as if it were streaming out behind you from the force of your leap.

Lift the crown of your head. Create maximum length in your spine. Breathe comfortably.

Releasing the Pose

To come out of the pose, exhale, lower the arms, take the weight on your hands again, and switch sides.

Variation

Embodying the Pose

Place a mat on the floor, and place a couple of bolsters or folded blankets across the mat. Place a single-fold blanket on the floor beyond your mat (not on the mat, because you will need to slide the blanket).

Kneel on your right knee, and draw your left heel to the front edge of the bolster or the stack of blankets on the mat beneath you. Take your hands to the bolster or blanket on either side of your hips.

Exhaling, stretch your right leg back, so that the kneecap to the toes rests on the floor. The knee will be slightly bent. The topmost part of the front of your right thigh, up to the groin, will rest against the edge of the bolster.

Stretch the left leg forward, taking the left heel to the single-fold blanket. Keeping the weight on your hands, exhale and slide the left foot forward until the left knee almost straightens. The back of the left thigh should rest against the front edge of the bolster.

Work both legs evenly. Draw the front sit bone back and the rear sit bone forward to level the hips. Shift your weight from your hands to your legs and feet.

Exhaling, bring the hands to namaste in front of your heart.

On the next exhalation, raise the arms overhead. (If your shoulders are very tight, keep the hands parallel and lift evenly, or hold a yoga block between your hands. Press the palms into the block, and lift evenly.)

From the great lift of your heart and chest and collarbones, look up, keeping the back of your neck long. Fly!

Sustaining the Pose

Recall the two foundational *yamas* (ethical principles) of the *Yoga Sutra*: nonviolence and honesty. Be honest about how flexible your hips and shoulders are, and have the patience to go slowly and compassionately as you deepen the pose. Accept support as long as you need it. Even a practitioner with very open hips may like using a thin blanket under the base of the body, to bring additional awareness to the hamstrings and groin.

Releasing the Pose

To come out of the pose, exhale, lower the arms, take the weight on your hands again, and switch sides.

Reflection

Hanuman, half-monkey and half-divine, the superhero who lives from his heart, is Rama's greatest devotee. In this story, he is the key figure in reuniting Rama and Sita because his extraordinary physical gifts, plus his love and faith in Rama, make him invincible.

Where do you strive in this pose? In your eyes, your tongue, your neck, your breath, your legs?

Can you open your heart when you are striving? Can you give 100 percent effort while at the same time offering the results to God?

How important is it to you to "get it right"? Does your desire to do your best ever slide over into perfectionism? When you are in perfectionist mode, can you also be compassionate with yourself and others?

Hanuman is fairly sure that Sita is on the island, but not sure where; he must leap across the ocean, over unknown territory, to find her. Has your intuition ever led you to make a leap into the unknown in search of some precious goal?

For a few breaths, rest your awareness in your heart, as Hanuman did when he carried Rama's ring to Sita. Feel the love and commitment that a hero needs; it's not all about strength.

My teacher liked to say that Sita symbolizes the mind, or individual consciousness, which should always be united with the heart. Sita becomes vulnerable to abduction when she is distracted by the charming golden deer. If we think of Sita as the part of us that gets abducted by the demands and distractions of the world, we can also see her rescuer, Hanuman, symbolically. Here, Hanuman represents the faith and the yoga practices that pave the way to the meditative reunion of our mind and spirit: asana and pranayama.

As the son of the wind, Hanuman can be understood to represent, above all else, the power of pranayama, which harnesses the mind and emotions with the breath of the body; and his role in Rama's story is very much involved with themes of linking, bridging, and reuniting.

If Rama is taken as a symbol of the *atman*, or soul, and Sita as a symbol of the mind, we can understand their separation as a state only too familiar to most of us. In this state, our attention is stolen, as it were, by the distractions around us, and we lose connection to our spiritual life. We become so involved with people, places, and things that we never seem to find time for our meditative and devotional practices. How often have you lamented that you wish you could meditate or have a regular asana practice, but it is so hard to find the necessary time—the space—the quiet? And you don't want to do it poorly; you want to give it your full attention and devotion. So ultimately you don't do it at all. But then you are left with a feeling of incompleteness, of missing something important and precious. This is the state of Sita, separated from Rama.

The breath mirrors our mental and emotional states. Quick, high, shallow breathing usually indicates pain, fear, anxiety; smooth, deep, long breathing tends to reflect a calm, steady state of mind and body, as in deep meditation or sleep. If we want to transform our state, the breath is an ideal medium. "Take a deep breath," we say to someone who is upset. If they follow our suggestion and continue breathing deeply and smoothly, soon they will calm down. When we learn practices to refine and direct the breath, particularly when the object of that practice is a steadier, more conscious connection with our spiritual ideals, then we are tapping into Hanuman's power, as the son of the wind, to reunite Sita with Rama.

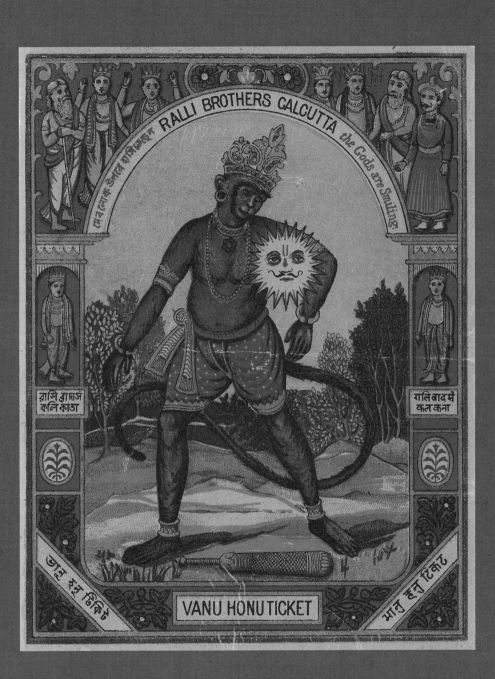

Hanuman captures Surya, the sun god.

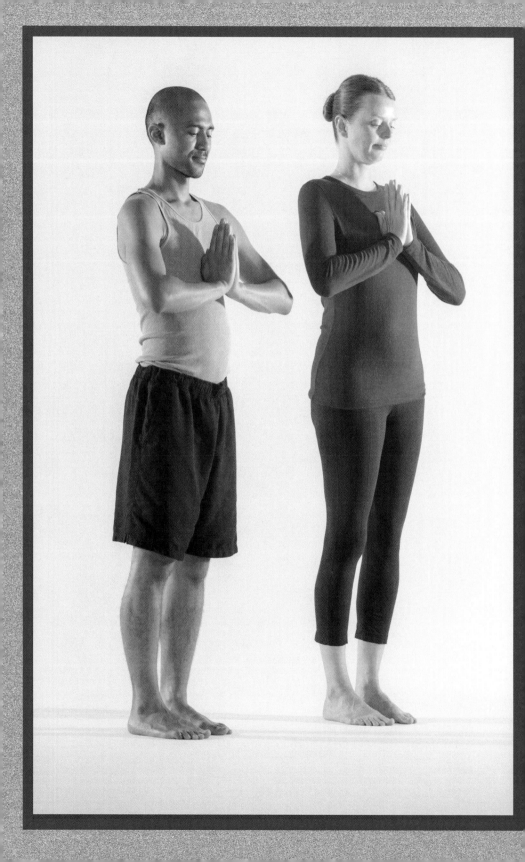

Hanuman Pays His Teacher's Fee
Sun Salutation / Surya Namaskara

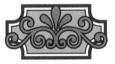

Hanuman was fascinated with Surya, the sun god, almost from birth. As a baby he saw the sun in the sky and mistook it for a high-growing, luscious fruit. Even as an infant, Hanuman had supernatural strength. Pushing off from the earth with his powerful monkey legs and stretching his long monkey arms, he leapt and soared to seize the sun—and succeeded. He popped it into his mouth. When Hanuman began to eat the sun, of course the universe went dark, alerting the gods that something was very wrong; and, of course, it scalded his mouth, but that stubborn monkey held on until Lord Indra hurled his diamond thunderbolt (*vajra*) straight at Hanuman's jaw. That did it: Hanuman opened his mouth and dropped the sun, and the universe's light returned. But that vajra hurt him; in fact, it broke his jaw, giving him the nickname "the one with the broken jaw," by which we know him today (*hanu* means "jaw"). The gods temporarily suspended Hanuman's powers. But because they were sorry about his jaw (although not about saving the sun), they also gave him special powers of strength, speed, shape-shifting, a gift for celibacy, a prodigious memory, and the qualities of a true lover of God, all of which would be restored to him in the future, when he would meet and serve Lord Rama. In the meantime, though, Hanuman needed an education.

The student-teacher relationship lies at yoga's heart. It is through our teachers that we learn the way to liberation. In Vedic times, the relationship between *shishya* and *guru* (student and teacher) was quite intimate, almost familial—a very different model than we have today, wherein yoga students can sign up online for a training, pay through PayPal or with a credit card, and then complete that training in a fixed period of time. In Vedic times, a student lucky enough to be accepted by a chosen teacher would live in that teacher's ashram until the teacher said they were done. The student-teacher relationship was literally priceless; but when the student completed his studies, he owed the teacher a fee (*guru dakshina*). This might be money, but usually not; it was a gift, a service, and it could be anything the teacher asked.

From ancient times, human beings have employed symbols for the ultimate teacher. One of the most enduring symbols is Surya, the sun. The beautiful Vedic prayer known as the Gayatri mantra addresses the sun as the one who illuminates our mind. Swami Vivekananda's English translation says, "We meditate on the glory of that Being who has produced this universe; may He enlighten our minds."

Since Hanuman was so fascinated with Surya, his mother, Anjana, made a suggestion: "Why not ask Surya to be your teacher? He drives his chariot all over the world every day and sees everything, everywhere. He knows all the sacred scriptures, and he flies even higher and farther than you can. I'm sure he has forgotten all about that little fruit incident when you were a baby." So Hanuman asked Surya to be his guru.

Surya refused. He had forgiven Hanuman for trying to eat him but said, "I have a strict schedule, no spare time at all. I must keep moving. I can't stop to teach you, and how can you learn effectively when I am moving? You can't."

"What if I keep up with you? Will you take me as your student then?"

"You won't be able to, but all right."

Hanuman flew up and positioned himself face to face with Surya, and Surya—who appreciated persistence in a student—began to speed across the sky, expounding scripture as he went. Naturally this meant that Hanuman was always traveling backward, with his face to his teacher, but isn't that as it should be? You shouldn't turn your back on your teacher; it's rude.

Hanuman was so dedicated that he mastered all the Vedas within a week. "What teacher fee may I offer you?" he asked Surya.

Surya—who was perhaps a little relieved to see him go—declined any payment. "Watching a devoted student learn is its own reward," he said.

"Well then," said Hanuman, "I can only offer you my gratitude and *namaskaras* [respectful greetings]." And so the sun salutation (*surya namaskara*) was born as Hanuman's guru dakshina to Surya.

Sun Salutation / *Surya Namaskara*

The salutation to the sun (*surya namaskara*) is a series of twelve asanas which are practiced as a flow. There are many, many variations and adaptations of this popular practice, and it would be impossible here to discuss all the creative possibilities. Some people jump from one position to the next. Some people do the whole series in a chair. The following version is the one I learned at Ananda Ashram, in 1964, from Sita Frenkel, a student of Swami Shivananda, at the beginning of my life with yoga (a version I still use today, with only slight variations).

Embodying the Pose
1. Stand in mountain pose (*tadasana*), with your weight evenly distributed through your feet. Join your palms over your heart.
2. Inhaling, separate your hands and sweep your arms up over your head. Stand with straight elbows, palms joined or facing each other; try to position your arms alongside or even behind your ears. Lift your chest, ground your heels.
3. Exhaling, sweep the arms down, folding at the hips, and touch the earth in a standing forward bend (*uttanasana*).
4. Inhaling, bend your right knee and bring your hands to the floor on either side of your right foot, fingertips aligned with the tips of your toes. Extend the left leg back, as in a runner's lunge. Your front knee should be at no less than a 90-degree angle—keep the

knee over the ankle or behind the ankle. Open your chest forward. Lower both hips toward the floor. Stay for a breath or two.

5. Exhaling, lift your hips and step your right foot back in line with the left foot, hip's width apart. Shift your weight back, lengthening your arms and your spine and keeping your sit bones high as you reach your heels toward the floor in downward-facing dog (*adho mukha shvanasana*). You may find that your heels don't reach the floor yet; if so, simply rest your weight on the balls of your feet.

6. Exhaling, and keeping your arms straight and strong, bring your hips down and forward until your torso is in a straight line from your head to your heels. Now you should be on the balls of your feet; reach your heels back and the crown of your head forward in downward-facing plank pose.

7. Exhaling, bend your knees and elbows. Touch your chin, chest, and knees to the ground. Keep your hips and buttocks up. This position is sometimes called six-point pose because all that touches the earth is your two hands, two knees, two feet, your chest, and your chin.

8. Inhaling, slide forward into cobra pose (*bhujangasana*). Bring your hands, palms down, in line with your shoulders. Peel your shoulders off the floor, draw your shoulder blades into your back, and lift your chest without altering the position of your neck. Lift with your back rather than pushing up with your hands. Keep your elbows bent and the back of your neck long. Press your legs and hips into the floor, and lift your spine.

9. Exhaling, put weight on your hands, lift your knees, and move your hips up and back until you are, once again, in downward-facing dog (*adho mukha shvanasana*).

10. Keeping your hands where they are, inhale and step your left foot forward between your hands in a runner's lunge.

11. Exhaling, bring the back leg forward, place your palms on the earth, straighten your knees, release your head toward the floor, and you are back in standing forward bend (*uttanasana*).

12. Inhaling, lift from the hips back to mountain pose (*tadasana*), keeping the spine long and sweeping your arms up overhead. Exhaling, lower the arms and join your hands over your chest. If this is the end of your sun salutation practice, then lower your arms and stand for a few breaths in mountain pose (*tadasana*). If not, then inhale, sweep your arms up, and repeat the sequence.

Reflection

This story has two aspects. The first is the one about baby Hanuman mistaking the sun for a luscious fruit and popping it into his mouth, causing the universe to turn dark, and his mouth to burn.

Consider: Have you ever misjudged a situation or a person, as baby Hanuman misjudges the sun? What happens when we leap impulsively for a goal that is not what we think it is? Think of a time when you were determined to go for something important—maybe a job or a relationship—that looked to you like a luscious mango, when in fact it was something larger, hotter, and more indigestible than you had imagined. Did anyone try to warn you of your mistake? Did you listen? What did it take to break the hold of the supposed "fruit" on your imagination? Were you hurt in the process? Did you receive any unexpected gifts as a result? Do you think that your mistake was spiritually significant?

The second aspect of this story is about the teacher-student relationship and how Hanuman offers the sun salutation (*surya namaskara*) as his teacher's fee (*guru dakshina*) to Surya, the sun god.

Historically, the sequence of poses we know as surya namaskara may have developed from an early sunrise practice that honored Surya as the source of energy and light for the world by greeting him with twelve of his most auspicious names and prostrating toward him.

In the 1920s, the Raja of Aundh introduced a fixed series into the schools of his tiny kingdom (now part of Maharashtra). He also published a small book urging every man, woman, and child to adopt this practice for the sake of their physical and spiritual health. Today, most yoga students learn some version of this practice early in their studies.

As you move through your surya namaskara, imagine facing your teacher—and not just any teacher, but your ideal, the one who guides and illuminates your life and universe as Surya does for the world. Offer each movement with love and gratitude.

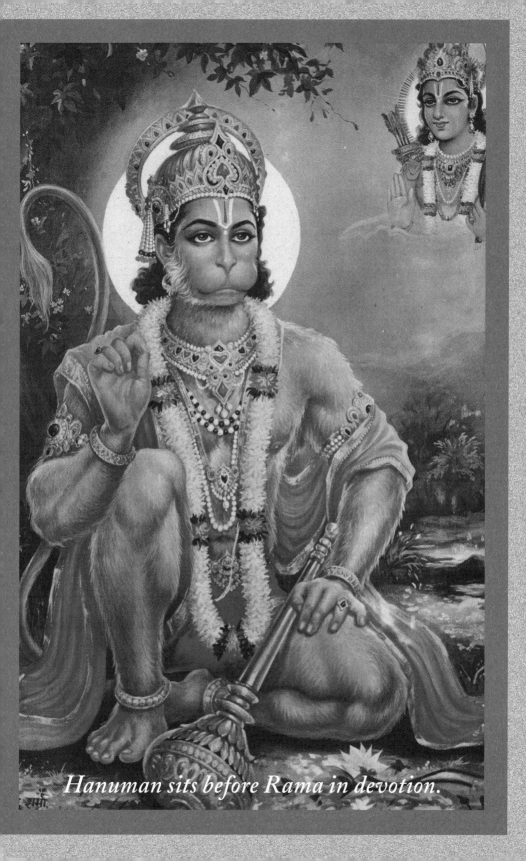

Hanuman sits before Rama in devotion.

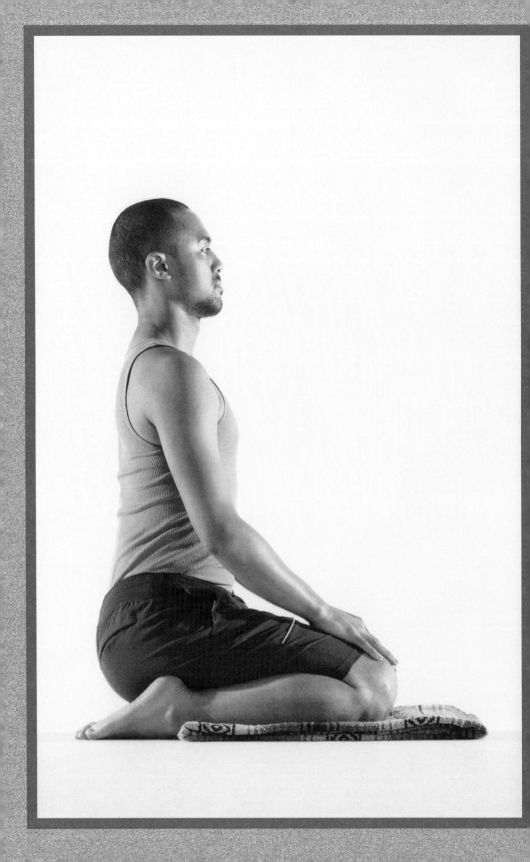

Hanuman the Hero
Hero Pose / Virasana

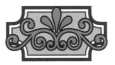

The verb *vir*, in Sanskrit, means "to subdue, to overpower, to tear open, to display heroism." Its related noun, *virya*, means "power, strength, energy, bravery, virility, manliness." *Vir* comes from a proto-Indo-European root, the dictionary tells us, giving it cognates in such seemingly diverse languages as Old Irish, Latin, Gothic, Hindi, and of course, English.

One of Hanuman's nicknames is Vir Hanuman (Hero Hanuman). He is said to have two primary attributes: *dasa* (servant) and *vira* (hero). In relation to Lord Rama, he is both. Some images of Hanuman emphasize his vira aspect: he leaps, he flies to the sun, he carries mountains, he performs impossible feats of strength and energy. But one of his most characteristic poses, one which shows his dasa side, is the one known by yoga students as the hero pose, *virasana*.

In this position, Hanuman kneels at Rama's feet. Sometimes he has one foot on the floor in front of him, sometimes he sits between his feet. In both cases, he demonstrates an attitude of devotion and service to a higher power; for Hanuman, Rama is not only the king, but the Lord incarnate. Hanuman's virasana puts his power, strength, and energy—his virya—in context.

Hero Pose / *Virasana*

There are many variations of *virasana*: twisted, forward-bending, reclining, half virasana. We'll do full virasana (shown in the photo) and half virasana. You may find it helpful to have some props near you, such as a folded yoga blanket and blocks, to ease strain in the knees, ankles, or feet. Stretching the ankles and feet in virasana regularly, over time, can create arches in flat feet and relieve the pain of heel spurs.

Full Pose

Embodying the Pose

Begin virasana by kneeling on the floor with your feet about 18 inches apart. Then sit between your feet, not on your feet, keeping the thighbones parallel. Place your feet just outside your hips, by the sides of the thighs. Let the toes point straight back. Rest the tops of the feet on the floor. Spread your toes. Rest your hands on your knees.

Modifications

If your front ankles are too tight for you to sit comfortably with the tops of your feet on the floor, place a folded blanket under your shins, letting the feet extend beyond the blanket's edge. Alternatively, place a blanket under the feet, ankle to toes. Some people enjoy elevating their feet, while others prefer elevating their shins to make space in the front ankles. The point is to find a position in which the feet can be active and alive in their relationship with the floor.

Sustaining the Pose

Pressing the shins and tops of the feet into the floor, lift your ribs and spine. Draw your shoulder blades onto your back. Imagine a line from the tip of each shoulder blade to the center of the collarbone on the same side; breathe back and forth along that line; sense the connection between the back and the front. Feel the shoulder blades supporting your collarbones and sternum. Breathe slowly and mindfully.

Remember Hanuman, and imagine a long, flexible tail extending behind you. If your tail feels restricted, sit higher. You can lower your props systematically as you gain flexibility.

Releasing the Pose

To exit virasana, shift the weight to your hands and swing your legs forward into the staff pose (*dandasana*). It's important to straighten your legs and "reset" the knees before proceeding to other poses.

Half Hero Pose / *Half Virasana*

Half virasana offers an interesting opportunity to observe asymmetries in your body.

Embodying the Pose

Sit with one side in virasana, as described above. On the other, bend your knee and place your foot flat on the floor, toes pointing forward.

Ground both sit bones. Are they level? Extend your tail. Press both feet down and lift your spine.

Place your hands in namaste position. Sit. Breathe.

Change sides and repeat the pose.

Sustaining the Pose

Compare sensations in the two sides. Do you need less support on one? Is one ankle tighter than the other? What degree of release or holding do you notice in each hip crease? Does one side of your rib cage lift more freely than the other? Let the freer, easier side show the more restricted side what is possible.

Where is your sense of ease, of rest, in this position? Where does the pose feel effortful? Do you tense your eyes or tongue in response to some sensation of gripping in the legs?

Take full virasana one more time, mindfully enlisting sensations of rest and alertness equally on both sides.

Releasing the Pose

When you release the pose, take time to breathe and enjoy any insight the pose has brought you.

Reflection

This story is about Vir Hanuman, relaxed and alert, equally a devotee and a warrior, surrendered at the Lord's feet, but ready to serve at any moment.

In *Yoga Sutra* 2:48, Patanjali tells us that by mastering postures, we become free from the afflictions of opposites (*dvandva*). By remembering Hanuman in virasana, we get a taste of the state in which the body's calmness frees the mind from its physical preoccupations. Once you have found the appropriate setup, virasana is an ideal position for seated pranayama or meditation.

In *Yoga Sutra* 1:20, Patanjali speaks of five essential qualities that help even ordinary people overcome obstacles in practice and in life: faith, vigor, retentive power, stillness of mind, and intuitive wisdom. The first two—faith (*shraddha*) and vigor (*virya*)—are intimately connected. Shraddha is the joy we take in our practice, the thrill of realizing its connection to the purpose of life. Shraddha leads naturally to virya: enthusiasm and energy for the practice, for realizing our potential to heal and transform our lives.

Vir Hanuman is a perfect example of integrated shraddha and virya. His loving faith in Rama is the source of his power and all his motivation. When he uses that vigor to serve his highest ideal, he can transform his body—for example, flying over the ocean and shrinking himself to a tiny size, in order to find and rescue Queen Sita—and alter events to serve the highest ideal.

Buddhist art depicts benevolent deities such as White Tara in the posture of "royal ease"—seated at a slight height with one leg drawn up into a bound-angle position, the other hanging down with the foot on the floor. This posture declares that she is both relaxed and fully prepared to come to the aid of her devotees at any moment. To me, half virasana has a similar energy: simultaneously grounded and laden with potential. One side of your body is a resting warrior, while the other is ready to respond.

Ask yourself: What do I love most, and what do I have faith in? What supports my efforts, and from where do I draw my strength? Write down some of the ways you see yourself being transformed by your practice. How has your practice helped you realize your ideals—physically, mentally, spiritually, interpersonally?

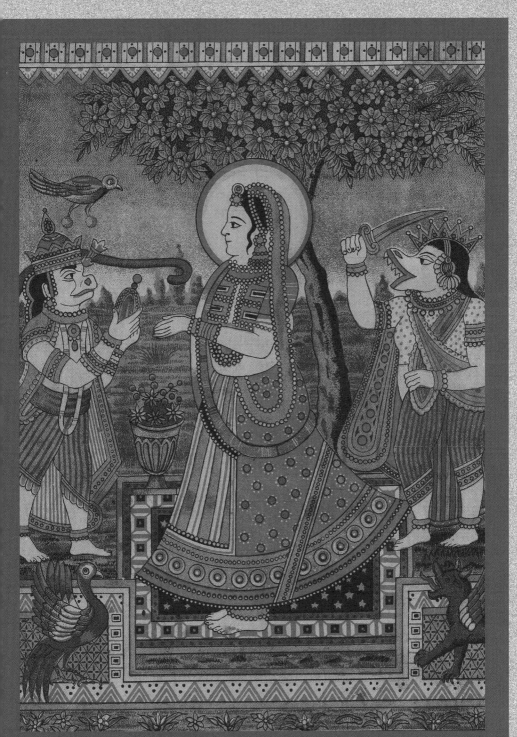

*Sita, captive under a tree, with
Hanuman showing Rama's ring and with
demon guard behind her.*

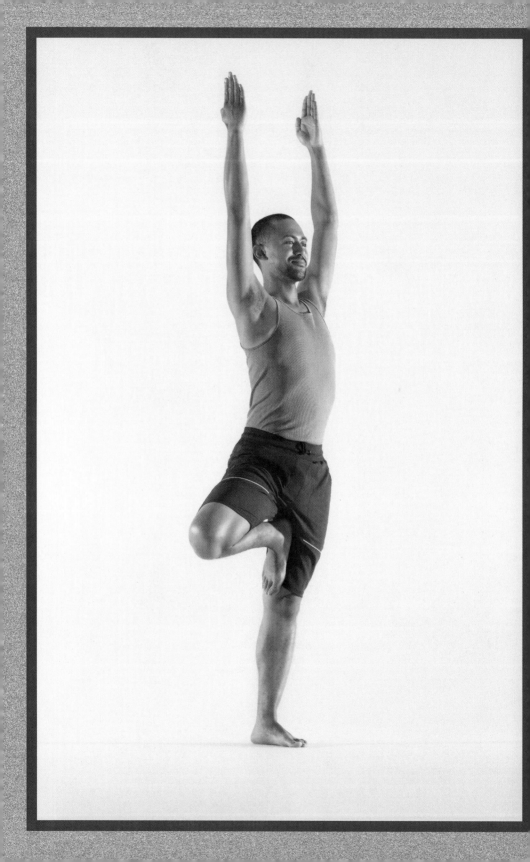

Sita in Captivity
Tree Pose / Vrikshasana

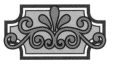

When Ravana took Sita to Lanka, he imagined at first that she would fall for him; other women did. He was handsome—once you got used to his ten faces—and strong and fabulously wealthy and powerful. His palace was a sensualist's dream of beauty and pleasant surroundings. Ravana was not unlike an urbane, highly influential drug lord—repellent and fascinating at the same time.

He offered Sita one pleasure after another, and Sita said no to it all. He proposed to make her his chief wife. Sita refused; she refused to spend even one night inside Ravana's beautiful palace. "I am your prisoner, not your guest," she said, "and I will never be your woman. Remember, I am Rama's wife, and he will find me. When he does, you will wish you had never seen me."

"I'm a generous man," said Ravana. "I will ask you every day to accept me. You have one year. After that, I will cook and eat you."

Outside the palace, inside its walls, stood a grove of Ashoka trees.

Ashoka means "without sorrow." Ashoka trees are symbols of love in Indian folk tradition. They are healers, containing powerful medicinal compounds. Sita lived under the trees, surrounded by Ravana's elite staff of *rakshasis*—monstrous women creatures with the faces of goats and fish and dogs, with hair sprouting from unlikely places and without the usual number of eyes and limbs.

The guards were ordered not to physically harm Sita, but they could use psychological methods to break her down. They told her that Rama would never find her, and even if he did, Lanka, being an island fortress and protected by magic to boot, was impregnable. They said that life in the comfort of Ravana's harem was a pretty sweet deal, as his hundred satisfied wives could attest. They said that a woman as beautiful, as royal, as Sita deserved to be treated like the queen she was and live in a palace, not wander the forest with her exiled husband. "Forget Rama," they said. "Think of all that Ravana can do for you. You're not leaving here alive anyway."

Sita sat with her back against a tree, and she breathed slowly, and she waited. She concentrated her mind on Rama. Every thought, every breath, every beat of her heart said, "Rama . . . here I am. Find me. Rama. Rama." She sent her love and longing into the trees and imagined their leaves broadcasting Rama's name to the atmosphere. Sita was the daughter of Bhumi Devi, the earth itself, and deep within she felt her kinship with rooted, growing things. Trees are patient creatures. They live a long, quiet time, and they know how to stand firm through all the changes of day and night, climate and season. Silently, those Ashoka trees spoke to Sita. "Stay still, little sister," whispered the trees with a rustle of leaves. "Be calm and steady, like us. Seasons change, we know, we know. This captivity is not forever. Stay still, and remember Rama."

On the mainland, Rama summoned Hanuman. "Go," Rama said, "find Sita. Don't frighten her! Take my ring. When she sees it she will know you come from me."

So one day, Sita heard a name called softly from above: "Rama, Rama." It was Hanuman, in the form of a tiny monkey. Hanuman spoke her beloved's name with all the love and longing that Sita felt in her own heart, and her heart told her to trust this peculiar messenger even before he produced a gold ring inscribed with "Rama-Rama-Rama" all around its circle. Hanuman's visit restored Sita's sense of connection with her Lord.

Tree Pose / *Vrikshasana*

The benefits of tree pose include improved balance and stability in the legs, feet, and pelvis—and the emotions. Practice this pose when life has you off balance, or when you have been moving too much. If your balance is of any concern, stand near a wall or a window ledge, which you can use to steady yourself, as needed.

Embodying the Pose

Begin by standing in mountain pose (*tadasana*) with your feet parallel and hip-width apart. Spread your toes. Lift your inner arches. Distribute your weight evenly between the right and left sides of your body. Settle your feet into the floor as if they were sending down roots.

Shift your weight to the left leg. Press down with the root of your big toe and your outer heel. Externally rotate your right leg and place the sole of your right foot on your inner left leg, above or below (but not on) your knee. Level your hips.

When you feel steady, stretch your arms overhead, hands parallel. Slide the shoulder blades down the back and release the shoulders away from your ears.

Sustaining the Pose

Imagine yourself as a tree in a grove; sense the calm, rooted presence of your tree companions. Gaze forward at a point that does not move. Widen your peripheral vision.

If you are near a wall, feel back through your body to sense its steady presence. Breathe slowly and quietly.

If your eyes tense or wander, or if your mind is agitated, your balance will waver. Be easy. Observe your mind, your breath. This pose may reveal unacknowledged distractions.

Can you draw stability from the earth?

Releasing the Pose

To come out of the pose, bend the elbows to the goalpost position and lower your arms to your sides; bend your left knee slightly and lower your right foot to the floor. Breathe and relax. Be aware of both sides of your body and how each side was affected by the pose.

Then repeat with the opposite leg.

Reflection

In this story, Sita, the feminine soul, is exiled from her beloved. She learns patience and equanimity through her deep connection with the earth, and her faith is renewed by connecting with her instinctive nature (Hanuman).

Trees appear throughout Indian sacred literature and art as symbols of the universe and as organic links between God and the individual. In this pose, imagine yourself as both Sita and the tree.

Sita, abducted and held captive, draws strength and comfort in nature. Contact with the earth helps her focus on Rama—who is, of course, not only her husband, but Lord Vishnu, a personification of ultimate reality. Her body may be constrained, but her mind is free.

Have you been in a situation where there was overwhelming pressure to accept a way of life or a set of values that fought with your own deeply held sense of what is right? What helped you to regain and maintain your equilibrium? Perhaps you were in a situation you couldn't leave when you chose; where did you find mental freedom? Did being in nature help?

The tree—patient, stable, and deep-rooted—offers protection to everyone who shelters beneath its branches, back snuggled firmly against its trunk. At the next opportunity, sit with your back to a tree and feel it breathe with you. Have you ever been called upon to comfort, to "back up" someone who needed your protection? Did their trouble disturb your equilibrium?

From my teacher's point of view, the *Ramayana* is filled with symbols. Sita is the mind, or individual soul, and Rama is the Lord, or cosmic soul. They are separated through the machinations of Ravana, the ego, who kidnaps Sita by tricking her into desiring a magical golden deer for a pet. The mind loses its focus on the Lord, the highest reality, and finds itself imprisoned. Now Sita must regain her meditative focus. What helps her? Remembering her Lord, being still and aware in a natural setting. What helps her even more, once she has begun that practice, is the appearance of Hanuman, her instinctive nature. As she gets more in touch with her body and senses, she realizes that Rama has been thinking of her all along.

When events like this happen in our lives, we sometimes call them coincidence or synchronicity. "I was just thinking of you, and you called!" Remember a time when you sincerely turned to God or to your practice for help, and suddenly the world seemed full of messages from the universe that you were on the right track. When that happens, you are Sita in the Ashoka grove, and those coincidences are Hanuman arriving with proof that Rama remembers you.

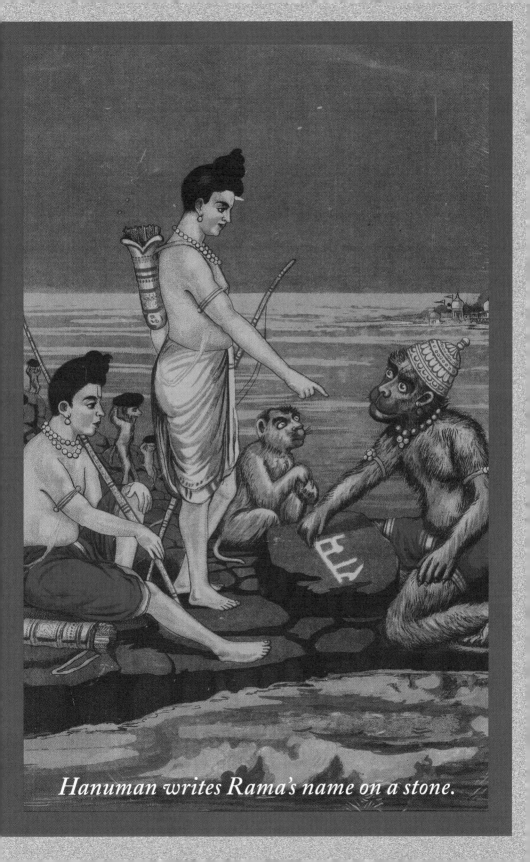

Hanuman writes Rama's name on a stone.

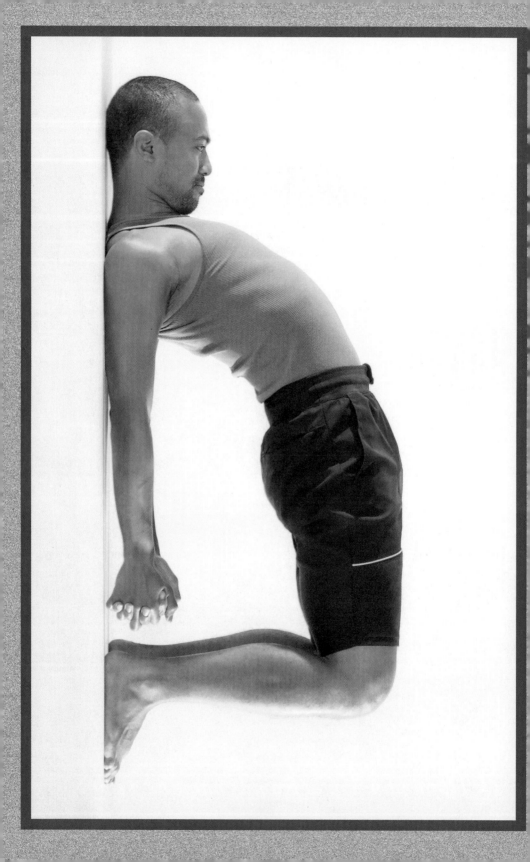

Faith Builds a Bridge
Bridge Pose / Setubandhasana

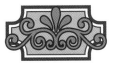

Once Hanuman had located Sita's prison on the island of Lanka, the challenge presented itself: how would Rama's army cross the sea to rescue her? Hanuman, son of the wind, could execute prodigious leaps and even fly, but the other animals and humans had no such powers. The distance from shore to shore was ten *yojanas*, eighty miles.

As it happened, among the troops was an engineer called Nala, the son of a Vanara woman and the celestial architect Vishvakarman, the "all-skilled." Nala set the army to the task of gathering giant boulders and timber, which they cast into the sea. But the boulders sank, as is the nature of boulders.

They stood on the beach, pondering. Hanuman was in the habit of writing Rama's name everywhere. It is said that Rama's name was even inscribed upon his heart. Lost in thought, with his finger he absently traced "Rama" on a half-submerged stone by the shore. To his astonishment, the stone rose to the surface and floated. Quickly,

Hanuman wrote Rama's name on more stones, and as he did, they became buoyant. This was the solution! Soon everyone wrote "Rama" on the stones, which floated in place obligingly. Within five days a solid causeway reached from the shore of India all the way to Lanka. Rama's army crossed the bridge, and the battle to free Sita began.

The demon king Ravana had once received a heavenly gift. This made him immune from harm by gods or other immortals—which, in his mind, meant he was unconquerable. Now his city was falling to an animal army—those very beings he had considered beneath notice— and Ravana himself was soon to lose his life to Rama, who, being born as a mortal, was not prevented by the boon from killing Ravana.

There is a sweet story about a ground squirrel that saw the bridge being built and wanted to help. He rolled in the sand, collecting grains on his coat, and then scampered to scatter the grains to fill in gaps between the stones. Some of the monkeys laughed at him and his minuscule efforts, but Rama was touched and pleased to see this tiny creature helping in his own little way. He picked up the ground squirrel in his left hand and stroked it gently, head to tail, with the fingers of his right hand. Even today, ground squirrels have three stripes down their little bodies to remind us how Rama loved and appreciated them.

Bridge Pose / *Setubandhasana*

There are several versions of bridge pose (*setubandhasana*), some active (shown in the photo), others more supportive and restorative. It is both a mild backbend and an inversion. How you express it and when you include it in your practice depends to a great extent on whether you want to emphasize its active benefits as a backbend or its calming qualities as an inversion. Let's look at both, starting with active setubandhasana.

Active Pose

Embodying the Pose

Lie on your back with your arms at your sides, palms facing down.

Exhaling, bend the knees one by one and place the soles of your feet on the mat. The centers of your heels should be in line with your sit bones. Make sure your feet are parallel and your shins are vertical.

Exhale as you press down through the four corners of the feet (roots of the big and little toes, inner and outer heels).

Exhaling, lift your pelvis. Roll the shoulders underneath you. Straighten your arms and interlace your fingers, palms facing each other. Ground your arms, pressing down into the floor from the tops of the shoulders through the outer wrists.

Sustaining the Pose

Elongate the spine, as if you could slide your pelvis toward your heels and your chest toward your head. Breathe quietly.

If you can reach your heels or ankles without compromising the vertical position of your shins, hold your heels or ankles. Feel how this variation lifts and opens your chest.

Releasing the Pose

On an outbreath, release your hands and lower the pelvis to the floor. Rest and breathe.

Repeat, clasping the hands with the other little finger on the bottom.

Supported, Calming Version

Embodying the Pose

Place a yoga block near your dominant hand.

Lie on your back, arms at your sides, knees bent with centers of the heels in line with the sit bones, shins vertical, feet parallel.

Keeping the head, neck, and shoulders on the floor, press into the feet, exhale, and lift the pelvis.

Place the yoga block under the sacrum at a comfortable height. Draw the tops of your shoulders to the floor. Lengthen the arms, palms up, reaching the tips of the fingers toward your heels.

Stay with bent knees for a few breaths. Then, one by one, slowly straighten the legs, keeping the centers of your heels on the floor. (If straightening the legs produces tension in the back, keep your knees bent and feel the weight on the soles of the feet, the block, and the shoulders.)

Clasp your hands so that the backs of the hands face the heels and the palms face the block. Lift and open your chest. Elongate the spine in both directions. Rest your weight on the heels, the block, and the tops of the shoulders.

Sustaining the Pose

When your knees are bent, your hips are probably going to be higher than your chest. When your legs are straight, the front of your body will be more level.

In either case, imagine that your heart is the highest point in the body. Feel the collarbones spreading like wings and the breastbone lifting and expanding.

Imagine that you can breathe through your heart center.

Releasing the Pose

When you are ready to release, let go of your hands. Have the knees bent so you can lift off the block by pressing into your feet and arms. Remove the block and lower yourself to the floor. Relax and breathe.

Reflection

In this story, a seemingly impossible task succeeds through the cooperation of unlikely allies in the service of a higher power and the common good.

Remember a time when your heart felt stony with grief or disappointment or anger. What helped transform it? Reflect, as you remain in this pose with your heart lifted and open: what name, what symbol, would be written on your heart to make it buoyant and strong enough to float? For Hanuman, Rama's name was powerfully transformative. What has transformed you?

Some people—Mahatma Gandhi, as one famous example—use Rama's name as their mantra. Try repeating it mentally, or softly, with the breath, as you exhale. See how this simple practice affects you. Does it lighten or open your heart?

A bridge, of course, is the connection and the path between two places, two states of mind or being, two people. A bridge may serve to connect our inner world with the outer world, our intelligence with our body, the individual with the Divine. Thinking symbolically, we can use this part of the story as a guide for reuniting our intelligence with the Self through mantra.

The sages say that the mantra is a name of the Lord, and sooner or later it will lead you to the Lord. The mantra is a bridge. Significantly, it is Hanuman, half-Vanara and half-divine, who discovers the power of Rama's name to align nature's elements in the service of divine union.

Notice that the army that rescues Sita is composed of animals—instinctive creatures not given to overthinking a situation. What does this mean to you? Is your body in touch with the instinctive wisdom that helps you regain the natural, integrated state we call yoga? Can you identify parts of yourself, your intelligence, that have been temporarily stolen? Has your feminine side been held captive by addictive or ego-driven behavior on your part?

No matter what "feminine" means for you, for our purposes here, consider defining it as some part of you that has been captured by addiction or oppression or socialization or trauma, an exiled part that needs to be reunited with your body, mind, and conscious intention. What does your body, with its instinctive, animal wisdom, know about reclaiming your soul? What parts of your life or personality have you discounted as powerless? Might they be the very aspects that can redeem you?

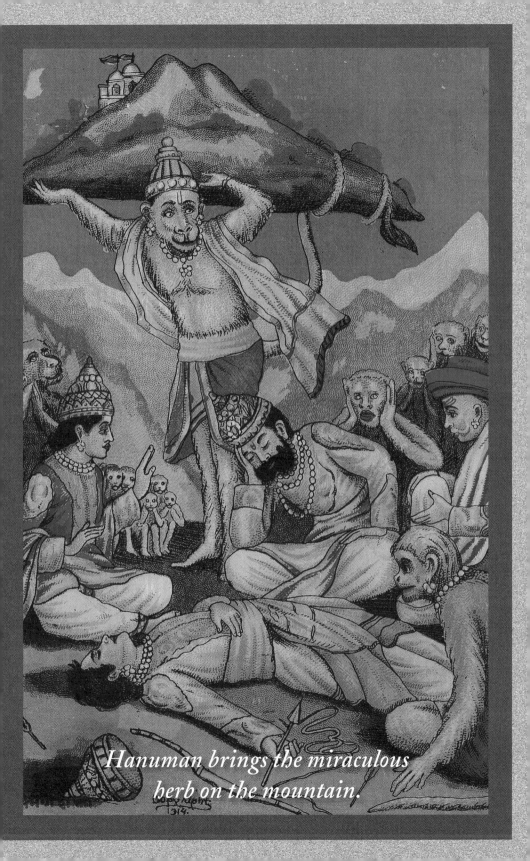

Hanuman brings the miraculous herb on the mountain.

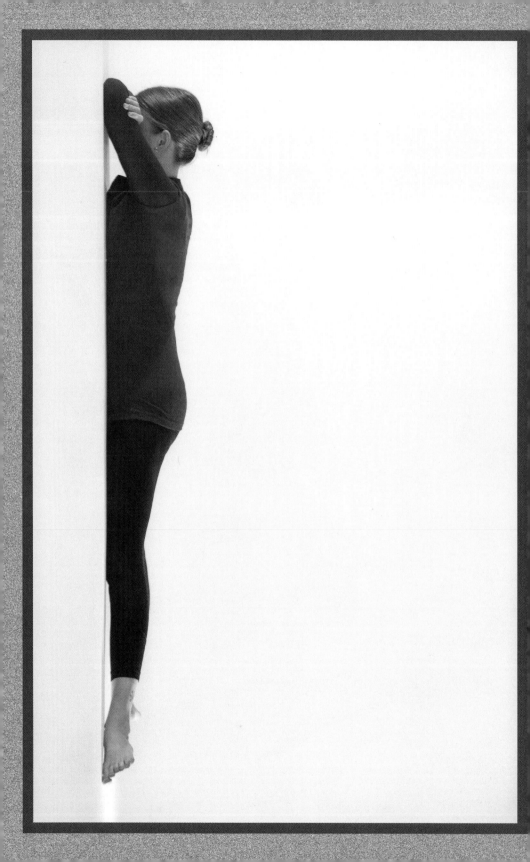

Attacked from Below

Crocodile Pose / Makarasana

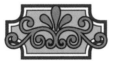

Once Rama's army crossed the bridge to Lanka, a terrible battle ensued. By the end of the second day, the field was littered with the bodies of the dead and injured. As the sun sank, Rama's brother Lakshmana lay grievously wounded, fated to die before the sun rose.

A Lankan royal physician knew of a miraculous herb native to a certain peak of the Himalayas, far to the north. Medicines prepared from this herb, it was said, could heal all hurts and even revive the dead. No one but Hanuman could possibly cover the distance and return before sunrise. "Hanuman," said Rama, "we need another of those leaps of yours. Go quickly!"

Hanuman leapt into the sky, over the ocean, and across the length of India. However, Ravana was aware of Hanuman's flight, and he sought the aid of his uncle Kalanemi to delay Hanuman's progress until after sunrise, or even better, to kill Hanuman himself. Assuming the guise of an ascetic, Kalanemi created the magical illusion of a hermitage on the shore of a lake, enticing Hanuman to stop and refresh himself. After praising the greatness of Rama, Kalanemi told Hanuman to go, drink deep, and cool himself in the lake's waters. "When you return, I will teach you a mantra for identifying medicinal herbs," offered Kalanemi kindly.

Hanuman flung himself gratefully into the cool water. But no sooner had he entered the lake than a monstrous *makara* (crocodile) seized him in its jaw and dragged him into the depths. Quick as thought, Hanuman became tiny, flew into the monster's belly, and then made himself huge, bursting its body as he escaped.

As he rose, spluttering, from the water, he beheld an exquisite *apsara* (a celestial nymph) hovering over the crocodile's corpse. "Son of the Wind," she said gratefully, "long ago, Ravana cursed me to be in crocodile form until I should meet the servant of Rama. Now the curse is lifted and I am free!" She revealed Ravana's plot to destroy Hanuman and Lakshmana.

As the apsara flew home to heaven, Hanuman quickly slew Kalanemi and continued on his journey. Finally, from the air, he could see Mount Dunagiri, "the Medicine Mountain," glowing. He landed, but he could not distinguish one healing herb from another. "No, no, I'm a monkey, not a physician! No time to waste. I'll just take the whole thing and let the experts sort it out." With that thought, he pulled the mountain up to the sky, set it on his shoulder, and began to fly south, speeding to Lakshmana's side, racing the dawn. And if Surya, perhaps, delayed his rising a little to help his former student, who could criticize him?

Crocodile Pose / *Makarasana*

Crocodile pose (*makarasana*) is wonderful for consciously using the diaphragm while breathing, and for relaxing the entire nervous system. The greatest benefits of this pose, which builds awareness and comfort rather than strength or agility, include relieving stress and low-back pain, gently stretching the paraspinal muscles, strengthening the diaphragm, and bringing awareness to the breath.

Embodying the Pose

Lie on your stomach. Place your feet slightly more than hip-width apart, with your toes pointing inward and heels outward. (For many people, this placement releases tension from the low back and creates a sense of spaciousness in the back of the lungs and diaphragm. If you find it awkward, just place your feet in a way that feels comfortable.)

Place your elbows in line with your shoulders; you can adjust the width for comfort. Fold your arms in front of you.

Press your elbows into the floor and drag your lower ribs forward, creating length in the side waist. Rest your diaphragm and lower front ribs on the floor.

Rest your forehead on your folded arms. Relax. (If you need more height under your head, use a folded blanket or a bolster; there should be no tension in your neck.)

Sustaining the Pose

Soften the root of your tongue, your throat, and your belly. Inhale and exhale all the way down to your tailbone.

Snuggle your front body into the floor like a crocodile luxuriating in the mud.

Breathe. Be in no hurry to go anywhere. Observe your breath and its movement in your body.

Notice, under the skin, the bony structure of your skull and ribs; feel down past the bone to the soft brain tissue and other organs that the hardness protects. Notice the softness of your belly in between the hardness of the lower front ribs and the hip bones.

Releasing the Pose

When you are ready to move on, simply roll to your side, bend your knees, and rest your head on your arm for several breaths. Push yourself to sitting and take a few more breaths before standing.

Cautions

Do not do if pregnant or if you have any condition in which abdominal pressure is uncomfortable.

Reflection

In this story, as Hanuman stops to rest, he is attacked by a hidden force from below the surface of the lake. By overcoming it, he is able to complete his mission on time.

The makara in Indian tradition is a fabulous beast, part crocodile, part elephant, sometimes part stag or peacock. It is the vehicle of the river goddess Ganga. Its name lives, transformed into *makar* in modern Hindi, as the name of the ordinary crocodile and in the name of the yoga asana, crocodile pose (*makarasana*).

The makara is associated with the second chakra. Located just above the tailbone, the *svadhishthana* chakra is associated with the water element, with the unconscious, and with deeply held emotion. The svadhishthana chakra is the seat of dormant *samskaras* (habit patterns, karmic impressions; see *Yoga Sutra* 4:9–11), whose unconscious hold must be released in order for you to realize your full potential.

In many healing rituals, you enter the water for renewal and purification, but in the water's depths you may encounter your personal demons. Just as a crocodile drags its prey under the water, your unconscious mind and its samskaras can grab you from below. Sometimes when people begin a breathing practice, they find things "coming up" from their unconscious in the form of dreams, memories, and long-forgotten emotions. This is because the breathing process is automatic, usually done unconsciously, and when you begin to make one unconscious thing conscious, others follow. This is part of the healing process; don't be deterred by what comes up. Stay with the practice, take refuge in the practice, and it will carry you through.

Hanuman saves himself by becoming bigger than the crocodile and bursting its hold. Spiritually, this could mean transcending your limits by aligning your consciousness with a higher, sacred power.

It is interesting that, in our story, Hanuman is flying on a healing mission when he pauses, comes down to earth, and goes to the water for refreshment. Something in the water (a complex?) threatens to drag him under, but he overcomes it, "bursting" through it, and continues his journey. In psychological terms, this resembles what happens when a person in a helping, healing role begins to be overextended and stops to ground herself. Finding herself confronted by personal issues she hasn't dealt with, she must first deal with them before returning to healing others.

Crocodiles symbolize the union of opposites. They have hard backs and soft bellies. Mother crocodiles carry their babies very gently in their powerful jaws, but they can also use those jaws to crush.

Crocodiles represent an equal balance between water and earth: they live in both elements and go easily from one to the other. Crocodiles have keen night vision. They see in the dark and underwater, but frequently remain unseen, due to their ability to submerge in the water and remain still in the mud, looking like logs—until they move.

As you breathe, remember a time when something unexpected "grabbed you from below." How did you break its grip? As a healer, when have you interrupted your helping journey in order to confront and resolve personal issues?

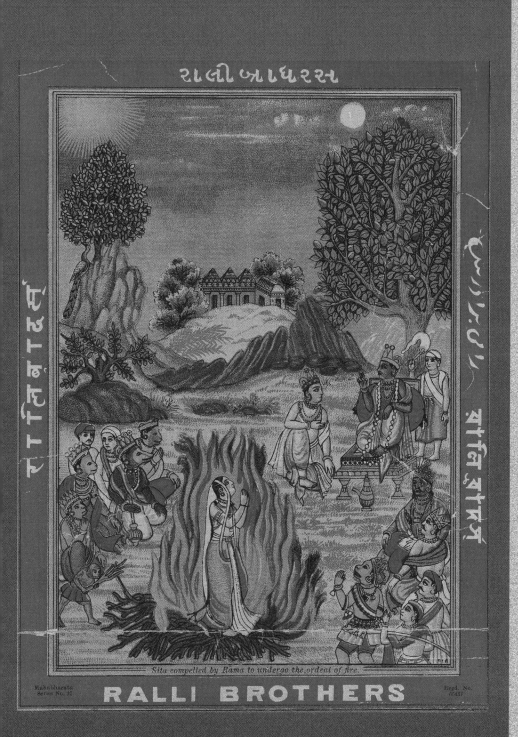

Sita compelled by Rama to undergo the ordeal of fire.

RALLI BROTHERS

Sita in her trial by fire for purity.

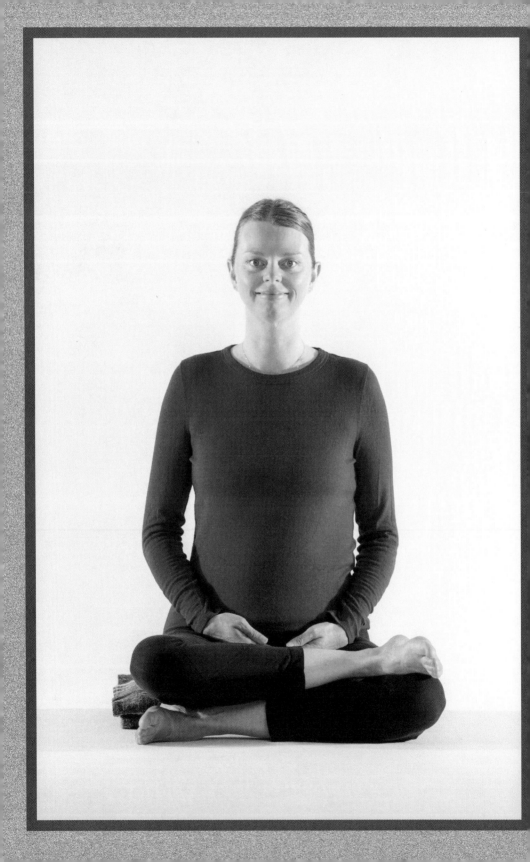

Sita's Trial by Fire
Fire Log Pose / Agnistambhasana

Once the battle of Lanka was won, Sita could not reunite with Rama until her purity was publicly established. Though not by her own choice, she had, after all, been a "guest" of Ravana for many weeks. Sita offered to prove her innocence through a fire ritual, and Rama accepted. Sita called Lakshmana to bring wood and construct the pyre. Their years in the forest had made Lakshmana an artist at starting fires. Calmly and without hurry, he selected good, aged, slow-burning logs and stacked them carefully, creating risers for the flames to climb to heaven. He sprinkled the branches with ghee and holy herbs. Sita circumambulated Rama with devotion and approached the fire with folded hands. "If my heart has been true only to Rama, let the god of fire protect me," she said. Then she fearlessly entered the fire.

The bright flames flew up, with a rush and a roar, and enveloped her. Through the brightness, the watchers saw the flames gather into the shape of a tall, shining man with robes of red and yellow: Agni, lord of fire, intermediary between earth and heaven. He gathered Sita in his sheltering arms. Turning to Rama, he said, "Please welcome back your pure and blameless Sita."

After honoring the fire, Rama joyfully took Sita in his lap.

Fire Log Pose / *Agnistambhasana*

Agnistambhasana resembles other seated poses such as *sukhasana* and *padmasana*, but in this pose the legs form more of a square than a triangle. Like those poses, this one provides a stable seat for meditation and seated pranayama. The physical benefits of fire log pose include stretching and opening the hips and groin, stimulating the abdominal organs, and calming the mind.

Embodying the Pose

To begin fire log pose, sit on a yoga block, or on the smooth edge of a small stack of folded blankets, with your knees bent and your feet on the floor, in a simple cross-legged position. Distribute your weight evenly between your right and left sides.

Inhaling, shrug your shoulders up, roll them back, and rest your hands on your lap. (If you feel a sense of drag in the shoulders, place a folded blanket across your lap to support your forearms and hands.) Lift all your ribs evenly.

Draw the navel in and up and lengthen your front body from just above the pubis to just below the sternum.

Slide your left foot under your right leg; place the little-toe side of your left foot on the floor. Begin conservatively, respecting the possible limitations of your knees by placing the left foot close to the right sit bone.

Now, use your hands to lift your right shin. Hold the right knee with your right hand and place your left hand under your flexed right foot.

Place the whole lower leg across, as one piece from knee to ankle, and stack the right ankle above the left knee.

Don't create a sickle shape with your foot: keep the outer edge of the right foot parallel with the floor.

Sustaining the Pose

Assess the stability of this foundation: How are your knees? If your hips are more flexible, work your bottom (left) foot forward until it is directly under the right knee and your shins are stacked parallel to the floor like two logs of wood. If this action strains your knee, keep the bottom foot back, closer to the right sit bone.

Is there space between the top knee and the foot it is resting on? If so, add support (a block or a blanket). Are both knees lifted off the floor? Maybe you need to sit higher or add blankets under both knees. Think of these props as the kindling material that helps your fire burn smoothly and brightly.

Press the outer heels down. Do you feel your hips opening?

Keep the feet active by spreading your toes. Do you feel your breath rising and chest lifting?

Let the crown of your head rise like the tip of a flame. Rest your arms and hands calmly in your lap.

Breathe. Fire is never static; the flames rise and fall. Watch your breath as if you were watching those flames.

Now, keeping the front body ascending, exhale and fold at your hip crease.

Reach your hands and arms forward along the floor in front of you.

Snuggle back your sit bones and lengthen the sides of the waist.

Soften the belly and tongue; enjoy the comforting sense of light pressure at the navel. Do you feel a stretch in the outer hips? Yes? Good, but respect any signs of strain in the knees.

Rest your arms and hands on the ground and, keeping your neck long and soft, relax your face.

Stay in the forward bend for a minute or so, longer if you are comfortable, breathing quietly and evenly.

Releasing the Pose

To come out, use the strength of your arms to lift the torso and uncross your legs. Repeat on the other side.

Reflection

In this story, Sita, falsely accused, prepares to sacrifice herself to establish her innocence. In the process she is exonerated.

The trial by fire serves two purposes: first, to publicly reunite Sita with Rama, and second, to demonstrate to the world the truth of her innocence. Rama and Sita, being deities, are here to help human beings transcend our limitations by modeling behavior that upholds dharma—the foundational values of humanity. When you have done nothing wrong but someone insinuates that you might have, it is very, very difficult not to get angry. Sita models keeping her temper; even in the fire, she is cool. She models not justifying herself, but leaving the results to a higher power—in this case, represented by Agni—for the sake of the people's peace of mind. Rama models solidarity by supporting her decision.

Have you ever been in a position like Sita's? Have you been the subject of accusations or insinuations about your behavior or motives? Have you witnessed someone else being accused? Consider how even false accusations can lead to terrible results for a community or a country. How can the firm, careful foundation and smooth, intentional breathing of fire log pose help in a situation like this?

In the *Rig Veda*, fire is personified as Agni (same root as our word "ignite"). Agni is said to be present in the fire of the sun, the stars, the lightning. He is in the digestive fire in our belly, and in the pillar of smoke that links us with the gods, and this world with the next. Agni, fire, is the agent of sacrifice and transformation. The sacred fire altar was a portal between the worlds, a threshold where prayers and sacrificial offerings could pass from earth to heaven, and blessings could descend from heaven to earth—all through the medium of fire (*agni*) and its logs (*stambha*). The ritual of building a fireplace was the centerpiece of ancient Vedic civilization, and many mythological stories feature fire and sacrifice—and the results of their correct or incorrect execution.

The Himalayan tradition teaches the path of *agni vidya*, the understanding that our own individual body is a vehicle of liberation. From this perspective, the body is a living altar of the sacred fire, and the physical world contains all the tools and means that we need to discover heaven.

Yoga practice is an art, just as building a fire is an art. For both, the foundation must be firm, dry, and well-situated; the logs and kindling—that is, your yoga mat and props—must be intelligently prepared and properly aligned. How might it change your practice if you approached each session as a sacred offering and an opportunity for transformation?

Ayurveda teaches that the digestive fire—also called agni—is located at the navel center; the gentle stimulation of this center through the forward bend in the fire log pose, coupled with deep, smooth breathing, helps us to assimilate and transform the fuel we consume as food and sensory input. What are you taking into your body? Physically? Emotionally? How does your practice help you to digest or transform it? Are there things your body does not easily accept?

The End of the Story

Reunited after Sita's trial by fire, Rama and Sita returned home to Ayodhya. All obstacles to Rama's kingship were gone. In a joyful celebration, Bharata removed his brother's sandals from the throne, where they had symbolically held his place all these years, and Rama himself sat in their place.

Valmiki says, poetically, that when Rama returned to Ayodhya, it was a moonless night, but Rama's presence illuminated the darkness. The people ran into the streets, rejoicing, carrying torches and lamps to light his way, and every house shone with lit, gem-encrusted lamps. Inner darkness was overcome: No one lied or stole or harmed another. Night-roaming predators remained in their lairs. The city was free of violence and discord. Petty conflicts and jealousies disappeared like shadows at noon.

For a time all was well and happy in Ayodhya; trees flowered and everyone behaved kindly. But eventually discord arose. It surrounded, of all things, Sita's purity. Evil-minded people whispered insinuations:

"She lived that long in Ravana's palace—do you really expect us to believe that nothing happened between them?" When Sita announced that she was pregnant, rumor insinuated that the child was not Rama's.

As king, Rama had to be a model of behavior for his subjects—a model of dharma. He knew he had to send Sita away, even though the rumors were unfounded. His subjects were whispering, "What kind of standards is our king upholding if he keeps in his house an impure wife carrying another man's child?" When people distrust their rulers, society suffers, dharma declines, and even crops and the weather go wrong.

Rama instructed Lakshmana to take Sita to the forest, near Sage Valmiki's ashram. Valmiki warmly welcomed her to the ashram, where she gave birth to twin sons. This gentle poet-sage secretly hoped to reunite Rama with Sita and her sons, and after several years, he composed the *Ramayana* and sent the boys to wander about the city singing it. When Rama heard about their beautiful singing, he asked them to sing at his palace. As they sang in the great assembly hall, all who heard them were entranced, and Rama and others of his family realized they were his sons.

Wishing to be reunited again with Sita, Rama immediately asked for her to be brought to the palace to take an oath before the assembly, testifying to her purity, to convince everyone of her innocence. Sita arrived at the assembly hall to take her oath, but she resolved that this would be the last avowal of innocence she would ever make—she would return to Mother Earth. In a clear voice, she called out, "Mother, if I have been faithful to Rama, take me home!"

The earth opened. From her depths there rose a throne, and on that throne sat Bhumi Devi, Mother Earth, garlanded with flowers, in a robe girdled by shining seas and rich with rivers. Opening her arms wide, she gathered her daughter onto her lap and enveloped her with her arms, as mountains embrace a smooth, green valley. The throne sank underground. The earth closed.

Rama grieved for Sita but continued to rule well and wisely for many years. Then, with his mission on earth accomplished, it was time for him to leave too. Bidding farewell to the people of Ayodhya, he walked into the waters of the river Sarayu until they met over his head. As Sita had taken the path of earth, he took the path of water, out of this world and into the timeless realm where myths originate.

When Rama left for the celestial realm, Hanuman stayed behind—Hanuman who loved Rama so much that Rama's name was written on his very bones. He asked for a favor: to be permitted to guard anyone who repeated Rama's name, so that no power in the universe could harm them; and he would be present wherever on earth Rama's story is told, whenever Rama's name is mentioned. And so he is. Under Hanuman's protection, all who hear Rama's story are blessed with health, joy, fulfillment, and wisdom; all who repeat Rama's name are transformed by it.

Rama and Sita's Journey Is Our Own

The *Ramayana*, like many fairy tales, tells the story of a young man, one who was meant to be a king, who had to give up his kingdom to wander in the wilderness. There he encountered demons and magical creatures. He befriended some of them. They in turn helped him to rescue his captive princess wife from the clutches of an evil magician, and regain his kingdom. Throughout the story both Rama and Sita behaved like ordinary human beings, subject to the limitations of time and space, although they were divine beings in fact. Rama was Narayana, Lord Vishnu; he had taken birth as Dasharatha's son in order to restore cosmic order and protect dharma. Sita was his eternal beloved, Lakshmi, the daughter of earth—creation personified.

To inspire us, Rama and Sita modeled a very human journey guided entirely by dharma and higher spiritual values. After meeting many challenges to their union, they returned home to the celestial realm, where they live eternally united.

The yoga tradition suggests that enlightenment for us is a similar journey, in which we must face obstacles and dismantle habits. We must give up the safety of our "kingdoms," our habitual sense of reality, to face the demons and magical beings that emerge in practice. We begin to recognize the separation between our inner Sita and our inner Rama, our mind and our heart, and we long for them to be eternally reunited. Creative engagement with myth helps reveal our self-created stories about who we are and how the world is. It helps us see what carries us away from a peaceful, purposeful, unified inner life and how, through meeting life's challenges, we can unite the scattered parts of ourselves into a lasting, fulfilling, and liberating wholeness.

Author's Note

You may have noticed that in some chapters of this book the details of the image in the text may vary from details in the narrative. That is because most of these images were never intended as illustrations for a particular written text. They *are* texts, recounting an episode from the point of view of a particular artist. They are visual approaches to a broader, sacred narrative that is common cultural property in a culture which, until quite recently, was largely oral and visual rather than written.

There are many, *many* versions of Rama's story, at least three hundred according to A. K. Ramanujan (see his article in Paula Richman's *Many Ramayanas*—listed in the Recommended Reading section at the end of this book). Not all of them are written. The best known and most widely recognized of the written texts are the ones by Valmiki and Tulsidas, and the *Adhyatma Ramayana*, a favorite of my teacher's. But there are feminist versions, versions in which Sita is Ravana's daughter, versions in which there are two Sitas and two trials by fire.

The sequence of events is by no means entirely compatible across versions. Did the trial by fire take place in Lanka, in Ayodhya, or both? Did Hanuman stop at the enchanted lake on his way to find the magic herb or on his way back? (And was that crocodile his daughter?) Since this is neither an academic work nor an effort to include every detail of the story, I have, in some instances, used poetic license to keep the story moving and to encourage readers to use their own creative imaginations in relating the stories (and images) to their own personal practice.

Bazaar Art

The images in this book represent the hybrid genre known as bazaar art, a blend of Western and indigenous art produced between the mid-nineteenth and mid-twentieth centuries. These inexpensive, mechanically reproduced icons of visual culture speak a common symbolic language to those who understand them. They include posters, trade labels, cigarette cards, and magazine illustrations. It is important to remember that these images were not intended so much as decorations as signifiers of important cultural and psychological realities embodied in India's sacred mythology.

Recommended Reading

Personal Practice

Goldberg, Natalie. *Writing Down the Bones*. Boulder, CO: Shambala Publications, 1986, 2016.

_____. *Wild Mind*. New York: Bantam Press, 1990.

_____. *The True Secret of Writing*. New York: Simon & Schuster, 2013.

Johnson, Robert. *Inner Work: Using Dreams and Active Imagination for Inner Work*. New York: Harper Collins, 1986.

Lasater, Judith Hanson. *Living Your Yoga: Finding the Spiritual in Everyday Life*. Boulder, CO: Shambala Publications, 2000.

Newell, Zo. *Downward Dogs & Warriors: Wisdom Tales for Modern Yogis*. Honesdale, PA: Himalayan Institute Press, 2007.

Translations

Buck, William. *Ramayana*. The Regents of the University of California Press, 1976.

Menon, Ramesh. *The Ramayana: A Modern Retelling of the Great Indian Epic*. New York: North Point Press, 2001.

Pant Pratinidhi, Bhavanrav Shrinivasrav, Rajasaheb of Aundh. *Surya Namaskars for Health, Efficiency & Longevity*. Aundh, India: Aundh State Press, 1940.

Rama, Swami. *The Valmiki Ramayana Retold in Verse*, Volumes 1 and 2. Honesdale, PA: Himalayan Institute Press, 1993.

Richman, Paula, ed. *Many Ramayanas: The Diversity of a Narrative Tradition in South Asia.* Berkeley, Los Angeles, London: The Regents of the University of California Press, 1991.

Tapasyananda, Swami. *Adhyatma Ramayana* (Sanskrit and English). Chennai, India: Sri Ramakrishna Math, 2006.

Tulsidas. *The Epic of Ram*, Volumes 1 and 2. Translated by Philip Lutgendorf. Cambridge, MA, and London: Harvard University Press, 2016.

Valmiki. *Mula-Ramayana.* Commentary by Shri Ramamurti. Monroe, New York: ICSA Press, Ananda Ashram.

Vilas, Shubha. *The Chronicles of Hanuman.* Noida, UP, India: Om Books International, 2016.

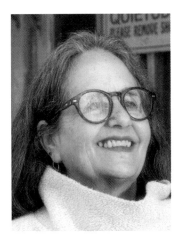

About the Author

Zo Newell, PHD, was introduced to yoga by the late Rammurti S. Mishra (Sri Brahmananda Sarasvati), MD, when she was fourteen. Other primary influences include Meher Baba, Judith Hanson Lasater, the Iyengar community, and Pandit Rajmani Tigunait and Sandra Anderson of the Himalayan Institute. She earned a doctorate in the History of Religion from Vanderbilt University, with a focus on modern Hinduism in written texts and visual images. Her first book, *Downward Dogs & Warriors: Wisdom Tales for Modern Yogis*, was published by the Himalayan Institute Press in 2007, and she has been a frequent contributor to Yoga International, with columns on mythology and yoga.

A former hospital chaplain and trauma counselor, Zo has taught yoga since 1991. She is a certified yoga therapist. She lives in Myrtle Beach, South Carolina, where she writes and teaches small classes and workshops on restorative work, therapeutics, and the personal uses of yoga's mythology and symbols. She is actively involved with an online writing practice community inspired by Natalie Goldberg's work. She has been married since 1981 to James R. Newell.

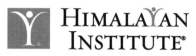

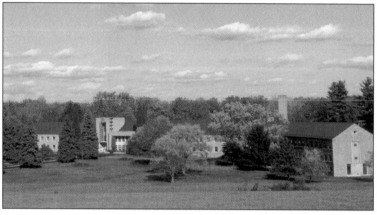

The main building of the Himalayan Institute headquarters near Honesdale, Pennsylvania

The Himalayan Institute

A leader in the field of yoga, meditation, spirituality, and holistic health, the Himalayan Institute is a nonprofit international organization dedicated to serving humanity through educational, spiritual, and humanitarian programs. The mission of the Himalayan Institute is to inspire, educate, and empower all those who seek to experience their full potential.

Founded in 1971 by Swami Rama of the Himalayas, the Himalayan Institute and its varied activities and programs exemplify the spiritual heritage of mankind that unites East and West, spirituality and science, ancient wisdom and modern technology.

Our international headquarters is located on a beautiful 400-acre campus in the rolling hills of the Pocono Mountains of northeastern Pennsylvania. Our spiritually vibrant community and peaceful setting provide the perfect atmosphere for seminars and retreats, residential programs, and holistic health services. Students from all over the world join us to attend diverse programs on subjects such as hatha yoga, meditation, stress reduction, ayurveda, and yoga and tantra philosophy.

In addition, the Himalayan Institute draws on roots in the yoga tradition to serve our members and community through the following programs, services, and products.

Mission Programs

The essence of the Himalayan Institute's teaching mission flows from the timeless message of the Himalayan Masters, including its founder, Swami Rama, and is echoed in our on-site and online mission programming: first we need to become aware of the reality within ourselves, and then we need to build a bridge between our inner and outer worlds. We seek to bring you the best of an authentic tradition, distilled for the modern seeker.

Our mission programs express a rich body of experiential wisdom, focused on yoga and meditation practice and philosophy, including our flagship Vishoka Meditation offerings. In-person mission programs are offered year-round at our campus in Honesdale, Pennsylvania, and include seminars, retreats, and teacher training certification programs.

The Institute is also a leader in hybrid in-person/online education. It offers a wide range of live online courses and certification programs, as well as on-demand digital courses. Join us in person or online to find wisdom from the heart of the yoga tradition, guidance for authentic practice, and a vibrant global community of like-minded seekers.

Wisdom Library and Mission Membership

The Himalayan Institute's online Wisdom Library curates the essential teachings of the living Himalayan Tradition. This offering is a unique counterpart to our in-person Mission Programs, empowering students by providing online learning resources to enrich their study and practice outside the classroom.

Our online Wisdom Library features multimedia blog content, livestreams, podcasts, yoga classes, meditation and relaxation practices, wellness content, and downloadable practice resources. These teachings capture our Mission Faculty's decades of study, practice, and teaching experience, featuring new content as well as the timeless teachings of Swami Rama and Pandit Rajmani Tigunait.

We invite seekers and students of the Himalayan Tradition to become a Himalayan Institute Mission Member, which grants unlimited access to the Wisdom Library. Mission Membership supports the Institute's global humanitarian efforts, while helping you deepen your study and practice in the living Himalayan Tradition.

Spiritual Excursions

Since 1972, the Himalayan Institute has been organizing pilgrimages throughout India and Nepal. Our spiritual excursions follow the traditional pilgrimage routes where adepts of the Himalayas lived and practiced. For thousands of years, pilgrimage has been an essential part of yoga sadhana, offering spiritual seekers the opportunity to experience the transformative power of living shrines of the Himalayan Tradition. Join us on pilgrimage in the Himalayas, or for retreat offerings at the Himalayan Institute Khajuraho campus in central India.

Global Humanitarian Projects

The Himalayan Institute's humanitarian mission is yoga in action—offering spiritually grounded healing and transformation to the world. Our humanitarian projects serve rural communities in India and Cameroon through education and literacy initiatives, health services, and vocational training. By putting yoga philosophy into practice, our programs are empowering communities globally with the knowledge and tools needed for a lasting social transformation at the grassroots level.

Publications

The Himalayan Institute publishes over 60 titles on yoga, philosophy, spirituality, science, ayurveda, and holistic health. These include the best-selling books *Living with the Himalayan Masters* and *The Science of Breath* by Swami Rama; *Vishoka Meditation, Sri Sukta,* and two commentaries on the *Yoga Sutra: The Secret of the Yoga Sutra: Samadhi Pada* and *The Practice of the Yoga Sutra: Sadhana Pada* by Pandit Rajmani Tigunait, PhD; and the award-winning *Yoga: Mastering the Basics* by Sandra Anderson and Rolf Sovik, PsyD. These books are for everyone: the interested reader, the spiritual novice, and the experienced practitioner.

PureRejuv Wellness Center

For over 40 years, the PureRejuv Wellness Center has fulfilled part of the Institute's mission to promote healthy and sustainable lifestyles. PureRejuv combines Eastern philosophy and Western medicine in an integrated approach to holistic health—nurturing balance and healing at home and at work. We offer the opportunity to find healing and renewal through on-site and online wellness retreats and individual wellness services, including therapeutic massage and bodywork, yoga therapy, ayurveda, biofeedback, natural medicine, and one-on-one consultations with our integrative medical staff.

Total Health Products

The Himalayan Institute, the developer of the original Neti Pot, manufactures a health line specializing in traditional and modern ayurvedic supplements and body care. We are dedicated to a holistic and sustainable lifestyle by providing products that use natural, non-GMO ingredients and eco-friendly packaging. Part of every purchase supports our global humanitarian projects, further developing and reinforcing our core mission of spirituality in action.

Residential Service Programs

Karma yoga (selfless service) is at the heart of the Institute's mission, and is embodied by the Himalayan Institute Residential Program and the SEVA Work-Study Program offered at our Honesdale campus. Learn more about residential service opportunities on our website, and join a vibrant community of practitioners dedicated to service.

For further information about our programs, humanitarian projects, and products:

call:	800-822-4547
email:	info@HimalayanInstitute.org
write:	Himalayan Institute 952 Bethany Turnpike Honesdale, PA 18431
or visit:	HimalayanInstitute.org

We are grateful to our members for their passion and commitment to share our mission with the world. Become a Mission Member and inherit the wisdom of a living tradition.

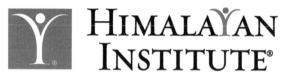

HIMALAYAN INSTITUTE®

inherit the wisdom of a living tradition today!

As a Mission Member, you will gain exclusive access to our online Wisdom Library. The Wisdom Library includes monthly livestream workshops, digital practicums and eCourses, monthly podcasts with Himalayan Institute Mission Faculty, and multimedia practice resources.

Mission Membership Benefits

Wisdom Library

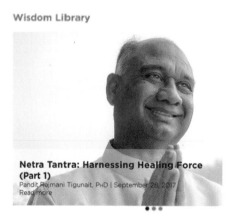

Netra Tantra: Harnessing Healing Force (Part 1)
Pandit Rajmani Tigunait, PhD | September 28, 2017
Read more

- **Never-before-seen content from Swami Rama & Pandit Tigunait**
- **New content announcements & weekly blog roundup**
- **Unlimited access to online yoga classes and meditation classes**
- **Members only digital workshops and monthly livestreams**
- **Downloadable practice resources and Prayers of the Tradition**

Get FREE access to the Wisdom Library for 30 days!

Mission Membership is an invitation to put your spiritual values into action by supporting our shared commitment to service while deepening your study and practice in the living Himalayan Tradition.

BECOME A MISSION MEMBER AT:
himalayaninstitute.org/mission-membership/

Downward Dogs & Warriors

Wisdom Tales for Modern Yogis

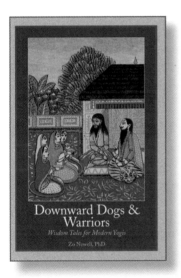

Have you noticed that colorful depictions of Indian gods and goddesses have made their way into the Western yoga scene, but are unsure how they can be useful in your personal practice? This book by a long-time yoga practitioner and scholar of religion provides an answer. It shows you how to use the physical postures of yoga along with deeply symbolic imagery for reflection, self-examination, and healing.

When I was young, my teacher told stories about Shiva and other heroes from the Indian epics. He explained that all the characters in the stories were aspects of our own minds, making the stories instructive as well as entertaining. For this book, I have chosen stories about Shiva related to well-known asanas in the hope that your yoga practice will be enriched and enlivened. I believe the postures themselves embody the energy of these stories, and I hope that knowing the stories behind them will help you to find the pose that emerges uniquely from your own body and from your own experience of yoga.
—Zo Newell, author

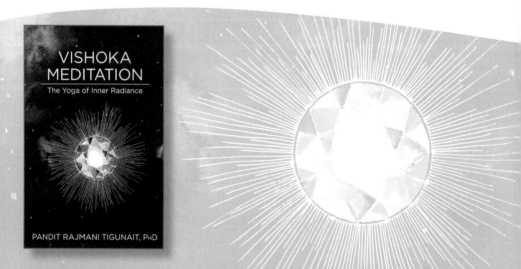
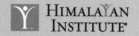

VISHOKA MEDITATION

The Yoga of Inner Radiance

Grounded in the authentic wisdom of a living tradition, the simple—yet profound—practice of Vishoka Meditation is the perfect complement to your existing yoga practice, as well as a powerful stand-alone meditation practice.

Learn Vishoka Meditation® Today!

- In-person Vishoka Meditation workshops at the Himalayan Institute and locations worldwide

- Online Vishoka Meditation webinars

- Vishoka Meditation teacher training certification program

- Vishoka Meditation immersion retreats, in-person and online

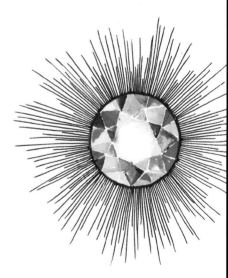

www.vishokameditation.org

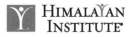

HIMALAYAN INSTITUTE

Sri Sukta

Tantra of Inner Prosperity

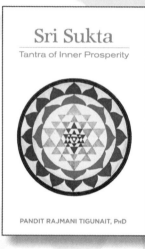

Sri Sukta—a cluster of sixteen Vedic mantras dedicated to the Divine Mother—is one of the greatest gifts to humanity given to us by the ancient sages. These awakened mantras empower us to pull the forces of abundance and nurturance toward ourselves so we can experience life's fullness.

Sri Sukta: Tantra of Inner Prosperity is the modern practitioner's guide to these mantras. Pandit Rajmani Tigunait's beautiful translation, commentary, and delineation of the three stages of formal practice help us unravel the mystery of Sri Sukta. This volume offers a rare window into the highly guarded secrets of Sri Vidya tantra—the heart of a living tradition—and reveals the hidden power of these mantras.

The wisdom of Sri Sukta is needed now more than ever. It holds the key to our individual peace and prosperity, and to a collective consciousness healthy and rich enough to build an enlightened society.

800-822-4547
shop@HimalayanInstitute.org
HimalayanInstitute.org

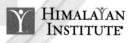
HIMALAYAN INSTITUTE

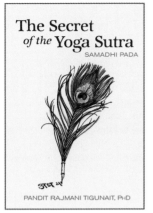

The Secret of the Yoga Sutra
Samadhi Pada
Pandit Rajmani Tigunait, PHD

The *Yoga Sutra* is the living source wisdom of the yoga tradition, and is as relevant today as it was 2,200 years ago when it was codified by the sage Patanjali. Using this ancient yogic text as a guide, we can unlock the hidden power of yoga, and experience the promise of yoga in our lives. By applying its living wisdom in our practice, we can achieve the purpose of life: lasting fulfillment and ultimate freedom.

Paperback, 6" x 9", 331 pages
$24.95, ISBN 978-0-89389-277-7

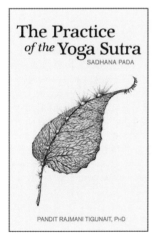

The Practice of the Yoga Sutra
Sadhana Pada
Pandit Rajmani Tigunait, PHD

In Pandit Tigunait's practitioner-oriented commentary series, we see this ancient text through the filter of scholarly understanding and experiential knowledge gained through decades of advanced yogic practices. Through *The Secret of the Yoga Sutra* and *The Practice of the Yoga Sutra*, we receive the gift of living wisdom he received from the masters of the Himalayan Tradition, leading us to lasting happiness.

Paperback, 6" x 9", 389 Pages
$24.95, ISBN 978-0-89389-279-1

800-822-4547
shop@HimalayanInstitute.org
HimalayanInstitute.org

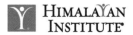 **HIMALAYAN INSTITUTE**

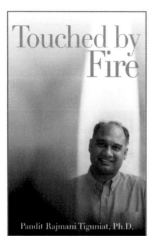

Touched by Fire
Pandit Rajmani Tigunait, PʜD

This vivid autobiography of a remarkable spiritual leader—
Pandit Rajmani Tigunait, PʜD—reveals his experiences and
encounters with numerous teachers, sages, and his master, the
late Swami Rama of the Himalayas. His well-told journey is
filled with years of disciplined study and the struggle to master
the lessons and skills passed to him. *Touched by Fire* brings
Western culture a glimpse of Eastern philosophies in a clear,
understandable fashion, and provides numerous photographs
showing a part of the world many will never see for themselves.

**Paperback with flaps, 6″ x 9″, 296 pages
$16.95, ISBN 978-0-89389-239-5**

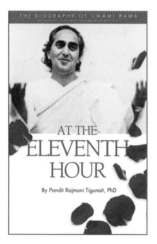

At the Eleventh Hour
Pandit Rajmani Tigunait, PʜD

This book is more than the biography of a great sage—it is a
revelation of the many astonishing accomplishments Swami
Rama achieved in his life. These pages serve as a guide to the
more esoteric and advanced practices of yoga and tantra not
commonly taught or understood in the West. And they bring
you to holy places in India, revealing why these sacred sites are
important and how to go about visiting them. The wisdom in
these stories penetrates beyond the power of words.

**Paperback with flaps, 6″ x 9″, 448 pages
$18.95, ISBN 978-0-89389-211-1**

800-822-4547
shop@HimalayanInstitute.org
HimalayanInstitute.org

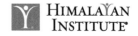
HIMALAYAN
INSTITUTE·

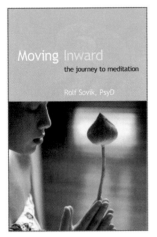

Moving Inward
Rolf Sovik, PsyD

Rolf Sovik shows readers of all levels how to transition from asanas to meditation. Combining practical advice on breathing and relaxation with timeless asana postures, he systematically guides us through the process. This book provides a five-stage plan to basic meditation, step-by-step guidelines for perfect postures, and six methods for training the breath. Both the novice and the advanced student will benefit from Sovik's startling insights into the mystery of meditation.

Paperback, 6" x 9", 197 pages
$14.95, ISBN 978-0-89389-247-0

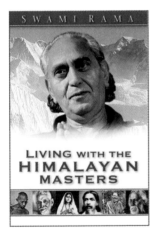

Living with the Himalayan Masters
Swami Rama

In this classic spiritual autobiography, hear the message of Sri Swami Rama, one of the greatest sages of the 20th century. As he shares precious experiences with his beloved master, Sri Bengali Baba, and many other well-known and hidden spiritual luminaries, you will have a glimpse of the living tradition of the Himalayan Masters.

This spiritual treasure records Swami Rama's personal quest for enlightenment and gives profound insights into the living wisdom that is the core of his spiritual mission and legacy. This living wisdom continues to enlighten seekers even today, long after Swamiji's maha-samadhi in 1996, sharing the timeless blessing of the sages of the Himalayan Tradition.

Paperback, 6" x 9", 488 pages
$18.95, ISBN 978-0893891565

800-822-4547
shop@HimalayanInstitute.org
HimalayanInstitute.org

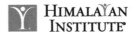

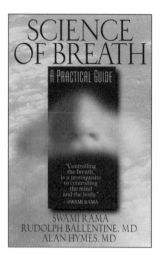

Science of Breath
A Practical Guide
Swami Rama, Rudolph Ballentine, MD, Alan Hymes, MD

People laughed at the image of pretzel-legged yogis focusing on the tip of their noses—until Swami Rama walked into a laboratory and showed scientists what a yogi with control over his respiration can actually do. Before astonished researchers, he demonstrated perfect control over his heart rate and brain waves—control physiologists hadn't believed humans could possibly achieve. In this book, Swami Rama shares some of the basic breathing techniques practiced by the Himalayan yogis so that we can begin immediately working with this powerful ancient science.

Paperback, 144 pages
$12.95, ISBN-13: 978-0-89389-151-0

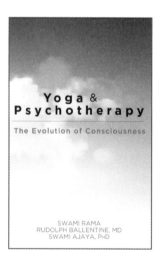

Yoga and Psychotherapy
The Evolution of Consciousness
Swami Rama, Rudolph Ballentine, MD, Swami Ajaya, PhD

For thousands of years yoga has offered what Western therapists are currently seeking: a way to achieve the total health of body, mind, emotions, and spirit. *Yoga and Psychotherapy* provides a unique comparison of modern therapy and traditional methods. Drawing upon a rich diversity of experience, the authors give us detailed examples of how the ancient findings of yoga can be used to supplement or replace some of the less complete Western theories and techniques. Offers an in-depth look at each of the seven chakras for the serious yoga practitioner and teacher.

Paperback, 305 pages
$15.95, ISBN-13: 978-0-89389-036-0

800-822-4547
shop@HimalayanInstitute.org
HimalayanInstitute.org

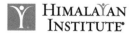

HIMALAYAN
INSTITUTE

Meditation and Its Practice
Swami Rama

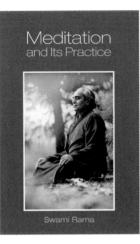

In this practical guide to inner life, Swami Rama teaches us how to slip away from the mental turbulence of our ordinary thought processes into an infinite reservoir of consciousness. This clear, concise meditation manual provides systematic guidance in the techniques of meditation - a powerful tool for transforming our lives and increasing our experience of peace, joy, creativity, and inner tranquility.

Paperback, 6" x 9", 128 pages
$12.95, ISBN 978-0-89389-153-4

The Art of Joyful Living
Swami Rama

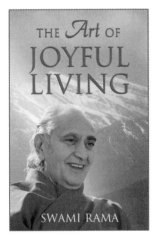

In *The Art of Joyful Living*, Swami Rama imparts a message of inspiration and optimism: that you are responsible for making your life happy and emanating that happiness to others. This book shows you how to maintain a joyful view of life even in difficult times.

It contains sections on transforming habit patterns, working with negative emotions, developing strength and willpower, developing intuition, spirituality in loving relationships, learning to be your own therapist, understanding the process of meditation, and more!

Paperback, 6" x 9", 198 pages
$15.95, ISBN 978-0-89389-236-4

800-822-4547
shop@HimalayanInstitute.org
HimalayanInstitute.org

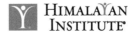

HIMALAYAN INSTITUTE

THE MUSCLE BOOK

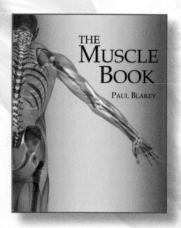

Paul Blakey, formerly an international ballet dancer and now a practicing osteopath, has written and illustrated this book for anyone who wants to know more about muscles.

The book clearly identifies all major muscles of the human body, and shows how they work. For each muscle there is straightforward information including common problems, signs of weakness, and self-massage for first aid.

Students of anatomy and physiology, yoga, massage, and dance, as well as athletes, will find this book to be an invaluable and easy-to-follow guide.

800-822-4547
shop@HimalayanInstitute.org
HimalayanInstitute.org

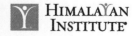
HIMALAYAN INSTITUTE